## *Praise for* The Unexpected Journey

———————

"Watching the journey our stepmom has bravely embarked on has been life-changing. Not only has she deeply educated and immersed herself in the world of caregiving, she has taken on this unexpected life change with poise and elegance. Emma's fierce devotion, endless compassion, and relentless quest to learn has been nothing short of extraordinary. Her care for our daddio is tender and unwavering, and the vulnerability she shares with the world is a lifeline for so many others walking a similar path. We are endlessly proud of her and profoundly grateful to be her family."

• RUMER, SCOUT, and TALLULAH WILLIS

"With grace, honesty, and unflinching courage, Emma has opened her heart to share the truth of caregiving—its heartbreaks and its hidden gifts. *The Unexpected Journey* is a lifeline for anyone navigating the complex world of dementia and it is her gift to every caregiver who has felt lost, overwhelmed, or alone. Through her story, Emma offers not just guidance but also the kind of empathy that only comes from living it."

• DEMI MOORE, actress

"This book is a game changer for caregivers of loved ones with dementia. It comes out of Emma's pain, which she has turned into a purpose bigger than herself. This book is brave, it's courageous, it's vulnerable, and it will change lives. I couldn't be prouder of her and the courage it took for her to write this. This will help millions of families, like hers, like yours, like mine, like everyone's. This is a must read, a must buy, a must give. It's a must. It's a book for our time."

• MARIA SHRIVER

"Becoming a caregiver to someone you love is one of the hardest and most heartbreaking jobs in the world, but Emma has documented her story with grace and empathy. From cover to cover, *The Unexpected Journey* is filled with straightforward, applicable information and honest reflections that will make every caregiver know that they are not alone."

• KATIE COURIC, award-winning journalist
and founder of Katie Couric Media

"Loving someone with FTD is a club no one wants to be a member of, but Emma has seized her moment to educate and create a community. Her advice and journey are meaningful and important for anyone, especially those thrust into the caregiver experience. A must read for anyone facing this challenge and seeking comfort, information, and humanity."

• JAKE TAPPER, CNN anchor and *New York Times* bestselling author of *The Devil May Dance*

"I admire Emma for telling her story of how strength, courage, and love can help you overcome fear and desperation in the face of neurodegenerative disease. Emma shares practical tips and valuable advice on how (and why) a caregiver can, should, and must take care of themselves. Giving of oneself and providing constant care for a loved one with dementia is beyond challenging, but *The Unexpected Journey* offers a road map forward on how to do so with balance and confidence."

• RICHARD S. ISAACSON, MD, preventive neurologist at the Institute for Neurodegenerative Diseases and founder of the first Alzheimer's Prevention Clinic in the United States

"Being a caregiver for a loved one with dementia—any kind of dementia—is a pilgrimage that none of us are prepared for. It can feel lonely and helpless. Emma learned the most important lesson: It doesn't have to be lonely, and you don't have to feel helpless. Reaching out to others, sharing the lessons that unfold every day, and listening to what others who have also been on that pilgrim's path have learned is some of the best work we can do on this earth." • PATTI DAVIS, author of thirteen books including *Floating in the Deep End*, daughter of President Ronald Reagan, and founder of Beyond Alzheimer's

"Emma's care partnering journey has been challenging, stressful, complicated, and beautiful at the same time—as most care partnering journeys are. With an unyielding determination to help others not feel alone in their experiences, Emma shares the many invaluable lessons she has learned so far. Her sincere advice and willingness to openly share her story are significantly helping to reduce stigma and improve the lives of those living with brain change and those who support them."

• TEEPA SNOW, MS, OTR/L, FAOTA, founder of Positive Approach to Care®

"I know from personal experience caring for my late mother that many of us step into the caregiving role without much preparation, and it can feel challenging and overwhelming. In *The Unexpected Journey*, Emma offers meaningful insight and practical advice that can help caregivers navigate this path with greater ease. A key message is that you can't effectively care for others without first caring for yourself. It is a powerful reminder for caregivers everywhere."

• JOAN LUNDEN, award-winning journalist, author,
TV host, and advocate for caregivers

"Emma's book is not just a practical resource—it is a lifeline for caregivers struggling with burnout, grief, emotional exhaustion, and the overwhelming sense of responsibility that often accompanies the role. We can all benefit from one of the most important messages in this book: Self-care isn't selfish—it's survival. Being a caregiver exacts a toll, and it's imperative that we carve out time for ourselves to reset and recharge. For anyone caring for an aging parent, a spouse with a chronic illness, or a child with special needs, *The Unexpected Journey* provides invaluable insights and important resources."

• TRACY POLLAN, actress and author

"*The Unexpected Journey* is the heartfelt guide every caregiver needs. Emma shares her powerful story with honesty and compassion, reminding you that while this road is difficult, you are never alone. This book offers wisdom, encouragement, and the reassurance that even in the hardest moments, there is hope, community, and a way to care for yourself while caring for someone you love." • DANIEL AMEN, MD, founder of the Amen Clinics
and author of *Change Your Brain Every Day*

"Having Emma as an advocate for our field is incredibly exciting because I think we're at a tipping point. People need to be aware of this disease, FTD, but they often don't hear it very well from scientists. Emma is really the first person of renown who has taken a step forward and shown the courage and willingness to speak out about this disease. Anytime anyone talks with Emma, they are moved, and this brings incredible hope to us in terms of raising awareness about FTD and the future of this disease. I can't tell you how grateful we are to her and her husband, Bruce."

• BRUCE MILLER, MD, the leading expert in FTD, distinguished professor of neurology at the University of California, San Francisco, and head of the Global Brain Health Institute

"Being a caretaker can feel like the loneliest and most isolated place. Because of the endless unknowns of neurological disease, there is so much that is needed but so little that is available. Emma took her pain and created a life raft of information for the many caretakers suffering in silence. We need to care for those who are caring for others with the same commitment. Emma has done just that." • SANDRA BULLOCK, actress and producer

"In her beautiful and heartwarming book, *The Unexpected Journey*, Emma combines her personal experience and insights from highly credentialed experts to offer advice that is helpful, relatable, and practical. Often a caregiver's last thought is to care for themselves, both physically and mentally, and this book guides you in very specific ways toward 'self-love' as you navigate loss and grief. No matter your age or experience or who you are caring for, this book is a welcome companion, ensuring that you grow on this journey."
• MARCIA GAY HARDEN, actress

"*The Unexpected Journey* is a deeply needed and beautifully written book for caregivers. Taking care of a loved one is not about having all the answers—it's about love, determination, and giving them the best quality of life possible. Caring for Tony [Bennett] was the most important thing I ever did, and though it came with challenges, it was also filled with moments of deep connection and meaning. Emma's book offers understanding, comfort, and wisdom to those on this journey, reminding caregivers that they are not alone."
• SUSAN BENEDETTO

"*The Unexpected Journey* is a testament to the healing power of storytelling. Emma's honest and heartfelt exploration of caregiving provides comfort, validation, and guidance to those walking this difficult path. Sharing our experiences—the struggles and moments of joy—helps us feel less alone and gives others permission to open up about their own journeys. This book is a gift to the caregiving community and beyond."
• LAUREN MILLER ROGEN, screenwriter, director, producer, and cofounder of Hilarity for Charity with her husband, Seth Rogen

"When a family member is faced with the immense challenges that a diagnosis like dementia brings, they unexpectedly realize they are the primary caretaker and often have no guidance or road map for how to proceed. They feel an overwhelming loss, anger, and fear as the world is crumbling around them. In

Emma's book, *The Unexpected Journey*, she offers a bridge to steadier ground. Through her candid explanations of her lessons learned as well as her research with the top doctors and experts in the field, she helps caregivers feel less alone and reframes the events that are happening to them so they can find ways to thrive even in the most unexpected and challenging times."

• M. NIGHT SHYAMALAN, writer and director

"When Emma stepped forward as a caregiver to her husband, it raised the profile of FTD families globally by putting a recognized and beloved face on this challenging disease. In *The Unexpected Journey*, Emma continues to elevate other families by shedding light on the needs of caregivers with grace and resolve. This book is a gift to every person who is on their own unexpected caregiver journey." • SUSAN DICKINSON, CEO of the Association for Frontotemporal Degeneration

"How brave Emma is to write a book about a journey that's all-consuming and terrifying, and ultimately beautiful. I wish that I would have had such a book to guide me. That would have been nice." • RON RIFKIN, caregiver

"Emma's big heart and unflinching honesty will be a blessed tonic for anyone struggling with how to attend to themselves as they attend to others. The single thing that makes sense about Bruce Willis being dealt this hand is that Emma has remained steadfastly by his side. Everyone who loves that man, myself included, owes her an endless debt of gratitude, and I know her readers will count themselves grateful, too."

• MARY-LOUISE PARKER, actress

"When a loved one is diagnosed with FTD, your entire world changes overnight—at least that's what happened to us when my father, Congressman Maurice Hinchey, received his diagnosis. But in these devastating moments, one of the strongest things anyone can do is turn heartbreak into action and hopelessness into community. Emma has done just that through her relentless advocacy and by sharing her own personal journey as an unexpected caregiver. Now with her book, *The Unexpected Journey*, she shares what she's learned with honesty and humility, creating a space for anyone navigating the difficult waters of becoming a caregiver and finding common connection through experience and insight."

• MICHELLE HINCHEY, New York State senator, 41st district

"Using the wisdom that comes from real-world experience, Emma weaves her own experiences as a caregiver, an understanding portrait of her husband's experiences as a person with dementia, and what she has learned from others into a readable and instructive resource for people caring for a loved one with dementia."

"I wish I'd had Emma's book to comfort and guide me when my husband was diagnosed with early-onset Alzheimer's and I had no idea what it meant or what lay ahead for me and my family. In *The Unexpected Journey*, readers will discover the power of healing, releasing shame, forgiving themselves, and embracing self-love and other emotions in the process. Priceless!"

"Emma is a bright, competent woman with extraordinary curiosity, eager to learn how to manage a situation that has no solution—her husband's dementia. Her book provides a treasure trove of information that she gathered for herself and others who are in the confusing and stressful position of caring for a loved one who has dementia. Through interviews and personal experience, Emma informs us all. I recommend her book highly, not just for primary caregivers, but also for their friends and relatives who may not understand the ambiguous loss of dementia. Emma's book is the best I have read for younger care partners, many of whom also have young children and even elderly parents to care for."

# The Unexpected Journey

# The Unexpected Journey

EMMA HEMING WILLIS

Finding Strength, Hope and
Yourself on the Caregiving Path

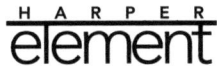

HARPER
element

HarperElement
An imprint of HarperCollins*Publishers*
1 London Bridge Street
London SE1 9GF

www.harpercollins.co.uk

HarperCollins*Publishers*
Macken House, 39/40 Mayor Street Upper
Dublin 1, D01 C9W8, Ireland

First published in the US by Open Field/Penguin Life,
an imprint of Penguin Random House, 2025

Published in the UK by HarperElement 2025

1  3  5  7  9  10  8  6  4  2

Designed by Christina Nguyen

A catalogue record of this book is available from the British Library

HB ISBN 978-0-00-872254-8
TPB ISBN 978-0-00-872255-5

Printed and bound in the UK using 100% renewable
electricity at CPI Group (UK) Ltd

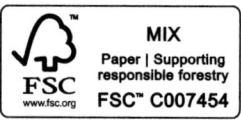

*To Mabel and Evelyn—my North Stars,*
*my guiding lights, my greatest teachers. Your well-being,*
*joy, and laughter are my compass, leading me forward even*
*when the path is unclear. May this book remind you that*
*even the hardest journeys can be faced with courage,*
*love, and a community to lean on.*

*To Bruce—the heart of my travels,*
*the echo in my footsteps, a love that endures beyond*
*every bend in the road. Your spirit is my constant*
*companion. I am forever grateful for you.*

*And to every care partner navigating*
*this unexpected journey—may you find solace in*
*knowing you are not alone, strength in a community*
*that surrounds you, and hope in the quiet moments that*
*whisper, You're stronger than you think.*
*This book is for you.*

# CONTENTS

# The
# Unexpected
# Journey

# Note to Readers

The information provided in this book, including insights from the author and contributing experts, is for informational purposes only and is not intended as medical advice. It should not be used as a substitute for professional medical guidance, diagnosis, or treatment.

Always consult your own physician or licensed medical professional, or that of the person you are caring for, before making any decisions regarding health care, including but not limited to medications, treatments, or daily routines. Any changes should be made under the supervision of a qualified medical professional.

This work is not intended to serve as a substitute for patient-specific professional medical guidance, diagnosis, or treatment. Medical and health-care decisions should be made only with focused professional guidance.

# Meet the Village

When my husband Bruce was diagnosed, we walked out of the doctor's office with nothing—no resources, no road map, no guidance on what to do next. I know many of you have been in that same traumatic position, left to make sense of an overwhelming new reality on your own. My hope is that this book can be a lifeline for you.

In the years since our diagnosis—yes, *ours*, because this is a family disease—I've built a network of trusted experts who have helped me become the best caregiver I can be. Their knowledge, wisdom, and support have been invaluable—not just for Bruce's care, but for my own well-being, too. Throughout this book, you'll not only hear parts of my caregiving story but also the voices of these experts, whose insights have made all the difference in my journey. My hope is that their guidance provides you with the same sense of support and reassurance, reminding you that you are not alone in this.

Daniel Amen, MD, founder of the Amen Clinics and author of several books, including *Change Your Brain Every Day: Simple Daily Practices to Strengthen Your Mind, Memory, Moods, Focus, Energy, Habits, and Relationships*.

Borna Bonakdarpour, MD, FAAN, FANA, associate professor of neurology at Northwestern University Feinberg School of Medicine, Department of Neurology, and cognitive/behavioral neurologist and investigator at Northwestern's Mesulam Center for Cognitive Neurology and Alzheimer's Disease.

Pauline Boss, PhD, professor emeritus at the University of Minnesota and author of six books, including *Loving Someone Who Has Dementia: How to Find Hope While Coping with Stress and Grief*.

Katie Brandt, MM, director of caregiver support services in the Frontotemporal Disorders Unit at Massachusetts General Hospital.

Danielle Cornacchio, PhD, clinical child psychologist and director of the WaveMind Clinic.

Diana Shulla Cose, founding executive director of Lorenzo's House.

Patti Davis, author of thirteen books, including *Floating in the Deep End: How Caregivers Can See Beyond Alzheimer's*, and founder of Beyond Alzheimer's, a support group for family members and caregivers of people with dementia and Alzheimer's.

Annie Fenn, MD, physician, chef, author of *The Brain Health Kitchen: Preventing Alzheimer's Through Food*, and founder of the Brain Health Kitchen cooking school.

Anne Front, LMFT, advanced palliative hospice social worker.

Nadine Gaab, PhD, associate professor of education at Harvard's Graduate School of Education.

Megan Graham, MS, certified child life specialist and vice president of research operations at Private Health Management.

Richard S. Isaacson, MD, founder and director of the Alzheimer's Prevention Clinic at Weill Cornell Medicine/NewYork-Presbyterian, the first of its kind in the United States, and director of research at the Institute for Neurodegenerative Diseases in Boca Raton, Florida.

Ty Lewis, an advocate, educator, and certified dementia practitioner who is her mother's caregiver.

Lauren Massimo, PhD, CRNP, FAAN, associate professor of nursing at the University of Pennsylvania and co-director of the Penn Frontotemporal Degeneration Center.

Bruce Miller, MD, the leading expert in FTD, a distinguished professor of neurology at the University of California, San Francisco, and head of the Global Brain Health Initiative.

Kathleen Murphy, MA, LMFT, a therapist in private practice who supervises monthly on-site workshops and founding chief clinical officer at Breathe Life Healing Centers in Los Angeles.

Kellyann Niotis, MD, director of Parkinson's and Lewy body dementia prevention research at the Institute for Neurodegenerative Diseases and its Parkinson's & Alzheimer's Research and Education Foundation.

Yolande Pijnenburg, PhD, professor of young-onset dementia at Alzheimer Center Amsterdam at Amsterdam University Medical Center in the Netherlands.

Habib Sadeghi, DO, cofounder of Entelechy Medical & Dental Community Center, an integrative health center based in Los Angeles.

Arlene Schollaert, MSW, LCSW, family services director of Amazing Place in Houston, Texas.

Bill Seeley, MD, professor of neurology and pathology at the UCSF Memory and Aging Center and director of the UCSF Neurodegenerative Disease Brain Bank.

Tali Sharot, director of the Affective Brain Lab in London.

Teepa Snow, dementia care specialist, consulting associate at Duke University's School of Nursing, and founder of Positive Approach to Care.

Wendy A. Suzuki, PhD, dean of the College of Arts & Science at New York University, a professor of neural science and psychology at NYU, and an internationally renowned expert in mental health and brain plasticity.

# Introduction

When we're in unfamiliar terrain, it helps to have a navigator—someone who can step in and chart a course through difficult landscapes, helping us face uncertainty with courage, find clarity amid confusion, and guide us along the way. But sometimes, life hands us situations where we become the navigator—thrust into the terrifying unknown without any warning.

When my husband, Bruce, was diagnosed with frontotemporal dementia (FTD), I suddenly had to lead the way on a journey with no map, no compass, and no sense of direction. At the appointment where we received the diagnosis, the doctor simply handed me a pamphlet—yes, just a pamphlet—and told us to check back in a few months. That was it. I was overwhelmed, frozen with fear, unsure of what to do or where to turn. To say I felt alone is an understatement.

What I really wished for was a road map—something to help me navigate this unknown with confidence and clarity. I needed more than medical information about Bruce's disease; I needed reassurance that, over time, I would find my footing. And I needed someone to tell me one of the most surprising truths of caregiving: The most important thing you can do for your loved one is take care of yourself. I've since learned that sustaining my own well-being is essential—not just for

Bruce, but for our two young daughters, Mabel (ten at the time of Bruce's diagnosis) and Evelyn (then eight), because they need me just as much.

Today, I've navigated a lot of that path (and I'm still navigating it), but it's taken time, energy, and resources, things I know not every family is fortunate to have. In this book, I'm going to share what I've learned so far, so that you have some guidance along the way.

First, some caveats. I'm not a doctor, a medical professional, or an expert. I'm not a specialist with all the answers, nor am I some enlightened care partner who knows how to caregive perfectly. I'm just a person—a mother and wife, traveling this journey with real emotions, in real time. I'm still very much in the thick of it, always bracing for the next shoe to drop. I'm doing my best to care for the husband I love deeply, while simultaneously raising our daughters, who are now thirteen and eleven.

What I'm sharing isn't in hindsight—I'm walking this path alongside you. I'm still learning, still going through it. Not a day goes by where life seems normal. In fact, I'm not sure I even know what normal looks like anymore. Some days, it feels like I'm trapped in a nightmare, waiting to wake up. My default state has often been worry, fear, anxiety, and catastrophizing—emotions that can take over if I let them. I've learned how to sit with these feelings, to acknowledge them without letting them consume me. Because of that work, I'm lighter now than I was in those early days when the siren in my head was on the highest volume. I've also found hope.

Over the past few years, recognizing that I needed to make this journey sustainable, I sought out and connected with some of the most trusted voices in the caregiving and dementia space. Their guidance, knowledge, and compassion have profoundly shaped the care partner I am today. The insights I've gained are priceless, and I knew I could not sit on this information and keep it to myself. Caregivers need all the support they can get, and that's how the idea for this book began to take shape.

Writing this book felt like an important way to pay it forward, something I know Bruce would be proud of because helping others was one of his core values. Sharing our experience is a way to honor him and offer you the comfort and guidance I wish I'd had at the start. My hope is that this serves as a kind of road map, one that empowers and grounds you as a care partner navigating this journey, bringing those aha moments to help light your path. More than anything, I'm sharing this part of my story so you feel the relief of knowing you are not alone.

I know some parts of this book may stir debate or feel triggering. People will have plenty of opinions, sometimes more opinions than actual experience. I'm also aware that some may feel I don't qualify as a "real" caregiver because I have the ability to hire outside help. I fully recognize the privilege of my position. Having professional caregivers is wildly different from doing this alone, without any support. I've walked both paths—especially in those early days when I didn't know what was wrong with Bruce and was too scared to tell anyone or realize that I needed help. No two caregiving journeys are the same. I know firsthand how uniquely challenging this path can be, no matter what it looks like.

I've witnessed how easily a caregiver's feelings can be dismissed or minimized simply because they have help. But caregiving is caregiving. Whether you have support or not, the emotional toll remains, and having support doesn't make the experience any less painful. My hope is that this book helps shift that narrative and brings more compassion into the conversation. It's vital that we stop comparing and competing with one another. What's most important is that we uplift and support the next caregiver who finds themselves in this role, whether it's by choice or circumstance.

THIS BOOK COMBINES my personal experience as a care partner with prescriptive insight into caring for yourself while taking on this difficult and emotionally taxing role. Before Bruce's diagnosis, I'd heard that metaphor that comes from the safety message flight attendants give right before a plane takes off: "In case of an emergency, put your oxygen mask on first before helping others." I thought it only applied to parenting, but I've since learned it is just as crucial when you are caregiving. I know your day is stressful and I know your day is hard. You're stretched and pulled in a million directions, but the truth is you can't care for your loved one unless you take care of yourself.

I learned this the hard way. With so much on my plate and so much uncertainty, caring for myself felt like the last thing I had time for. Nothing was more triggering—or easier to dismiss—than when someone would ask, "Are you looking after yourself, Emma?" I remember thinking, *How the hell do you expect me to do that?!* In retrospect, however, I wish I had prioritized taking care of myself sooner. It would have helped me think more clearly and feel less anxious and alone with the weight of the world on my shoulders. My hope with this book is that you'll see the value in it, too, and realize that checking in with yourself isn't selfish—it's self-preserving. None of this works if the caregiver is not cared for. This book is here to give you permission to prioritize your own well-being—something caregivers often struggle with.

———

ALTHOUGH MY STORY is FTD focused, this book is for anyone who is a caregiver to someone with any form of dementia. Those who are caregiving for people with other conditions may gain insight, too. Of course, not everything in this book will apply to you. But if you get even one nugget of information, one piece of insight, or one moment of comfort, then this book has done its job.

Recently, I watched a documentary called *Like Harvey Like Son* about an ultra-runner, Harvey Lewis III, who wanted to set a record running the Appalachian Trail, which is more than two thousand miles long and goes through fourteen states. The film shows Good Samaritans who leave snacks and cold drinks in coolers in places where hikers and runners are bound to come across them at some point. They call it "trail magic," and it gives the hikers and runners a boost and lets them know someone cares about them and believes in what they are doing.

I want this book to be that for you, some "trail magic" as you navigate your journey, because I care about you and I believe in what you are doing.

So what will you find in the chapters of this book?

- **Making Sense of the Changing Brain:** Dementia can feel overwhelming, and in this chapter you'll learn why gaining insight into what's happening helps you better understand your loved one's behavior. This clarity can ease acceptance, reduce stress, and allow you to plan for today and the future. For me, grounding myself in the reality of the situation was a vital first step that made moving forward feel more manageable.

- **Build Community and Connection:** Caregiving takes a village. Here I'll talk about how to surround yourself with others who are on a similar journey. This network can help you feel less alone and better understood and provide valuable insight and information from those who have been there. Community and connection are some of the best parts of this experience.

- **Make Time for Yourself:** In this chapter, I'll make the case that taking care of yourself is not optional; it's mandatory. (There are even studies that prove this.) It will make you a better care partner and is truly the only way you can travel this unchosen path without losing yourself mentally and physically. It's not selfish, it's self-preserving.

- **Focus on Your Brain Health:** As a dementia caregiver, you're at an increased risk of cognitive decline, so keeping your brain healthy is important. The good news is that it's never too late to think about your brain, and all the pillars of brain health benefit the rest of your body, physically and mentally. Implementing them is easier than you think. In this chapter, you'll find tips and guidance for focusing on your own brain health.

- **Expect an Array of Emotions:** Often caregivers are perceived as endlessly patient, selfless people who are admired as quietly heroic and unbreakably resilient. So when we have challenges and struggle with conflicting emotions, we view ourselves as bad people or failures. Here, we acknowledge that caregivers are human and all the emotions you feel—the good, the bad, and the ugly—are valid. I wish I'd known these things instead of beating myself up and feeling guilty or confused over my difficult emotions.

- **Parenting While Caregiving:** Caring for your person while raising children means you're doing two of the hardest jobs at once. This chapter highlights how to navigate this experience, whether you are part of the "sandwich generation" and caring for a parent and your own children simultaneously, or the person you're caring for is your partner or spouse. The behaviors that you model and the way you talk to your kids can greatly impact their experience.

- **Bringing In Help:** As you'll hear often throughout these pages, caregiving is not a solo mission, and at some point, you will need help. This doesn't mean you have failed your loved one; in fact, the most loving thing you can do is make sure your person's needs are met, which includes having some assistance so that you can go back to your special role in his or her life.

- **Let Friends and Family Take Care of You:** One difficult part about caregiving is the judgment, comments, and opinions you receive from other people, even those who are well-meaning. This adds more stress to a highly stressful job, especially because care partners tend to be so vulnerable and sensitive. Here we talk about how to handle this judgment and constant suggestion-giving. I provide a section written directly to your friends and family so you can educate them on the best ways to help you without you having to say a word.

- **Reframe the Journey:** While you didn't choose the dementia caregiving path, you can choose how to accept and reframe your experience, which is what we'll discuss in this chapter. As a result, you can uncover the positives that can emerge from something so challenging. I made a promise that FTD would not take me and our family down with it, and shifting my mindset has been one way to honor that. As much as I grieve this experience daily, just as I know so many others do, it has also revealed a strength I never knew I had. Our resilience isn't something to gloss over; it's something to acknowledge.

Throughout, you'll also find parts of my caregiving story with Bruce, not to sensationalize or fuel tabloid gossip, but because I believe in the power of personal stories to connect us and help us learn and grow from one another. Sharing builds camaraderie, hope, and inspiration, things that are vital for healing and moving forward. At first, I was hesitant to share my story in a book. But writing has allowed me to unburden myself and process so much of what I held inside for far too long. When I hear how someone else has triumphed over tragedy, it reminds me that I can keep going, even when the odds feel stacked against me.

The only way I can truly offer this perspective is through the lens of my experience with Bruce. That's why I'll start with our love story. While this part of the book may look different from your experience, it feels important to honor our love, honor our children, and begin from a place of warmth and affection, because that's where our journey started.

## A FEW THINGS TO NOTE

- Read this book in whatever way works for you. You can read it start to finish, or do so out of order, focusing first on the chapters that are most relevant to where you are in your journey. I've written each chapter so that it can stand alone. Also, feel free to make notes in the margins, underline passages (something I love to do when I read so I can go back to important info), and visit my website— emmahemingwillis.com—where I expand on some elements of the book.

- Also, you may find some ideas repeated multiple times. I've done this on purpose to ensure that you have comprehensive information in case you're reading the chapters out of order. Plus, I personally appreciate when key ideas are repeated and reinforced because life as a caregiver is overwhelming, and focus is hard to come by. If you feel the same way, I hope these reminders serve you well.

- I use the words "care partner" and "caregiver" interchangeably. Personally, I prefer "care partner," a term that resonated deeply when it was introduced to me by Teepa Snow, a dementia care specialist, consulting associate at Duke University's School of Nursing, and founder of Positive Approach to Care (PAC). She says:

While more people are familiar with the term "caregiver," we prefer to say "care partner." The reason for this subtle shift is the basis of our philosophy that we are supporting a person living with dementia. We are helping them do things or doing things *with* them; we don't do things *to* them. The relationship comes first, we are in this together, we are partners. We do what we do, ultimately, with their permission, in some form or fashion.

For me as a wife, becoming my husband's caregiver seemed to separate me from him, and I wasn't ready for that. I wanted to be a partner in Bruce's care. The term "care partner" continues to keep me close and aligned with him on our journey.

- You will also see that I use the terms "loved one" and "your person" interchangeably because Bruce is my loved one and my person. However, I acknowledge that not every caregiver is looking after someone he or she is close with. In fact, you may be caring for an individual you don't even like or with whom you have a complicated relationship, and that brings its own set of challenges. If this is the case, I know that the words "loved one" and "your person" might not resonate.

# ONE

# Bruce: A Love Story

Life is short. Live it to the fullest. Appreciate
every moment, every hour, every day, because in
the blink of an eye it may be all over.

**BRUCE**

Before I understood that Bruce's brain was changing because of a disease, I was mostly just confused. Thank goodness I knew who he was at his core; if I didn't, I don't know that I would have been able to stay in our marriage.

I can't pinpoint exactly when it started, it's very gray, but at some point, our relationship began to feel off. There were conversations that I recalled differently than Bruce did, and there seemed to be a lot of miscommunications between the two of us. Sometimes I'd think, *Is he for real? Is he pretending? Or am I going crazy?* The disconnect was subtle but happening more and more.

Eventually, my patience began to run thin. I was often annoyed with Bruce, yet I knew nothing was more important to him than me and our family, so I found his behavior puzzling. But he didn't mention anything was amiss and his doctors didn't flag any health concerns with me, so I assumed everything must be okay.

*Even if I* did *go to his doctor, what would I say?* I thought. *That I was noticing this abstract, intangible difference in my husband? Would they believe me or think I just needed a bitch-fest?* (I later learned that a lot of partners/spouses feel this way and it prevents them from talking to the doctor.) I couldn't really put what I was seeing into words myself, so how could I tell someone else? On top of everything, I was too scared to reach out to other experts or specialists for support because, of course, I wanted to protect Bruce and our privacy.

To say it was a difficult, confusing, and lonely time is an understatement.

Although I was uncertain about what was going on, one thing was clear: This wasn't typical Bruce behavior. Not only was he a high-performing, high-functioning person, but when we first met, Bruce was the take-charge one in our relationship, and I was happy to follow his lead. He made the plans and ran the ship of our lives. It's something I found attractive about him from the very beginning.

I MET BRUCE back in 2005 through my personal trainer, Gunnar Peterson. This was at the height of my modeling career, and Gunnar's legendary workouts at his home gym in Beverly Hills kept my body on point for that job. One day after my workout, I was walking to my car and saw Gunnar in the distance talking to two guys. I waved goodbye. Instead of waving in return, Gunnar yelled out.

"Emma, I want to introduce you to Bruce and Stephen!"

*Shit,* I thought. I was a hot, sweaty mess and not really in the mood to meet anyone new. But Gunnar was the ultimate connector, introducing everyone around him to one another. I had no choice but to walk over.

After a quick introduction, I shook hands with Bruce and Stephen Eads (one of Bruce's closest friends and his right hand) and then off I went. Was it love at first sight? No. Not at all. At the time, I was engaged. In fact, I didn't think much of the interaction. When Bruce and I later discussed that first meeting, however, this was his point of view: When I walked out of the gym, he looked at Gunnar and said, "Who is that?!" Then Gunnar called me over, made the introduction, which he would have anyways, and after I left, Bruce said, "I'm going to marry that girl one day."

Yes, Bruce's confidence was next-level!

Over the next six months, Bruce and I ran into each other often at Gunnar's gym because his training slot was right after mine on the Mondays, Wednesdays, and Fridays when I wasn't traveling for work, and from our brief conversations, I began to get to know him. Bruce was a nice, considerate, down-to-earth guy who was always curious and asked me questions about my life and career. His interest seemed authentic, never pushy.

One day, I told my mom about seeing Bruce at the gym.

"He's so nice and really attractive," I said.

"Emma! You're engaged to be married!"

"Don't worry, Mom. It's just an observation." The truth is, I wasn't a Bruce Willis fan per se. Yes, I grew up watching *Moonlighting* but had seen only one of his movies, *Armageddon*, when it first came out in the late '90s. Besides that, I didn't really pay much attention to him.

A few years went by. I didn't see Bruce much. During that time, my fiancé and I called off our engagement. He ran a few popular Hollywood nightclubs so perhaps that's why Page Six in the *New York Post* wrote about our breakup. I later found out that one of Bruce's longtime friends, Chris Sileo, had seen the article and told Bruce. That's when Gunnar called me.

"Can I give him your number?" Gunnar asked. "He's a really good guy and he's had a crush on you for years."

I agreed. I trusted Gunnar and already had a positive rapport with Bruce, so there was no downside.

When Bruce called me and asked me on a date, I told him the timing was off. This was the truth since I was in the midst of packing to move back to New York, had goodbye dinners scheduled with LA friends every night, and just wasn't in the headspace to go out on a date.

"I get it," he said.

The next day my phone rang. It was Bruce again.

"Listen, I understand you're very busy and you must be tired. But can I take you to get a tea?" he asked. "Also, I'm a strong guy. I can help you pack and move boxes."

He was persistent but charming, and I gave him so much credit for that. I was already having dinner with a friend that night and called her to see how she'd feel if Bruce came along. My thinking was this: At that time, Bruce's celebrity status meant he couldn't go out without paparazzi following him and rumors swirling. If he was seen out with two women, well, he'd look like the stud he was, but no one could make up a story about us dating. My friend understood and was fine with Bruce joining us.

So, was it love on our first date (if you can even call it a date)? No. The dinner was okay but definitely not a ten out of ten. Bruce seemed very nervous, bless his heart, and I felt off, too. I just wasn't in the dating mindset. Still, Bruce was a total gentleman from start to finish. At the end of the evening, he walked me to my front door, asked if he could give me a hug, and we said good night. That was a Friday, and on Monday, I moved back to New York City.

From there, Bruce and I started talking on the phone, at first a few times a week and then daily. Through those conversations I got to know him even more. And I started to like him. Actually, I *really* liked him. I loved how simple and humble he was, and there was something so nice about getting to know one another through long conversations—it was almost like being a teenager in high school on the phone for hours— very romantic and innocent.

During one of these calls, Bruce invited me to Parrot Cay, Turks and Caicos, for New Year's Eve, where he'd be celebrating with his three daughters, his ex-wife Demi, her then-husband, and some friends. Now, a trip with his children, ex-wife, and ex-wife's husband seemed like a lot to handle when we'd never really spent any time together. Plus, I'd already made plans with my best friend Ali for New Year's.

"I can't make it. But let's catch up when you come to New York in January," I told Bruce, who was bicoastal at the time.

"Why don't you just bring your friend?" he urged. "I'll send my plane to pick you up in St. Barts. You can stay with us and have your own private villa. Four bedrooms."

"That's so generous. Thank you," I said. "But our plans are cemented." I meant it and didn't even consider changing them. That is, until I told Ali about Bruce's invitation.

"Emma, are you nuts?" Ali said. "You play everything so safe all the time. You're single, he's single. This guy has been jumping through hoops every step of the way and you are declining his offer so you can stay in your comfort zone? He's sending us a jet, giving us our own villa, and his family is there. Clearly, his intentions are good. We are going, and you need to loosen the hell up!" *Yikes. Um, okay.*

If it wasn't for Ali, I would not have fathomed doing something that was so out of my comfort zone. But I did. So the two of us went to St. Barts for a few days and then Bruce's plane, *Jet Bruno* (or *400 Mike*, as he called it), picked us up on December 28. (I know, I know, fuel emissions, but this was decades ago. I also know it's extra, over-the-top behavior, but Bruce was always very extra. And it's part of our love story.)

When we landed in Providenciales, we were taken to the boat dock where Bruce was waiting to greet us, and he whisked us away to Parrot Cay. Once we arrived, he gave us a tour of the island on his golf cart. On our way to the house, we saw Demi. Boy, was I anxious.

"It's so nice to meet you," Demi said with the most welcoming smile as she gave me a hug, then Ali. *Phew.* That was one big exhale. Then we pulled into Bruce's beautiful compound and saw his three daughters, Rumer (who was eighteen at the time), Scout (then fifteen), and Tallulah (then thirteen). I'd never dated a man with children before, and this was the real cause of my anxiety. *What do they think of me being here?* I wondered. *Are they into it or will this be a source of stress?* I was a whole bag of nerves and silently cursed Ali for pushing us into this situation.

But as I got out of the golf cart with butterflies in my stomach, the girls greeted me with open arms. *Wide*-open arms and huge warm smiles.

"It's so nice to meet you, Emma. We've heard so much about you!" they said.

A second big exhale. (That initial encounter encompasses a glimmer of exactly who those three girls are as people: warm, kind, and accepting. I remember thinking that if I had kids one day, I hoped they would have the same lovely demeanor.) In the years that followed, I learned that the girls just wanted to see their dad happy. They knew having me there was giving him a sense of joy, so they welcomed it.

Up until that point, I knew Bruce in one way from the gym and another way from our long phone calls. That trip showed me yet another side of him: family man. Nothing was more important to Bruce than being a father, and his devotion to his three girls was something I'd never seen before. I didn't grow up with a dad who was present day-to-day like that. In fact, after my parents divorced, I went years without seeing my father. As I watched Bruce connect with his girls, I thought, *That's the kind of man I envision as the father of my future children.*

Bruce also made it a priority to have a good relationship with his ex-wife and her then-husband. Their cohesiveness was unconventional yet beautiful, and it was different from anything I had witnessed to date. *I can totally do this*, I thought. In fact, I *wanted* to do it. I wanted to be a part of a family that embraced unity and peace for the sake of their children.

Walking into Bruce's world taught me a new definition of family and friendship. Is it perfect all the time? Of course not, but it's human, refreshing, and full of love and respect. I'm eternally grateful to have it in my life. It's also something ingrained in our young daughters, Mabel and Evelyn. I'm proud they get to witness it and be a part of such a solid and connected blended family.

I left that trip, flew back to New York in love with Bruce, and the rest is history.

On March 21, 2009, we were married in front of thirteen friends and family members on Parrot Cay. Stephen, who was there the first time that Bruce and I met, officiated our marriage. After we said our "I dos," we all went over to the beach volleyball court to play a few fun and competitive rounds in our wedding outfits. Then we ate dinner under the stars, and because it was so small and intimate, each of our guests had the opportunity to get up and say something. There wasn't a dry eye at that table; mine and Bruce's were especially red and swollen. After the toasts, we danced, swam, laughed, and fed each other wedding cake until the wee hours of the morning.

To this day, it was by far the best party I have ever been to with only thirteen people.

OVER THE YEARS, I fell more in love with Bruce. It wasn't because of the big things, but rather all the little ones.

I loved how Bruce ordered food at a restaurant. He would get a wide variety of appetizers and entrees because he wanted us to try a bite of everything. I loved that anytime we got a bottle of wine with dinner, he'd have our waiter try a glass, too. "This way you'll know how to describe it to the next customer," Bruce would say. I loved that he understood the value of a good tip. "Always be generous," he'd say. "I worked in the service industry and relied on those tips." In fact, he was the most generous person I have ever met.

I loved that Bruce was a total gentleman. If I got up to use the bathroom at a restaurant, he would stand to see me out. And when I returned, he'd stand again to help me back into my seat. With Bruce, chivalry was not dead. I also loved how he supported the underdog. If a sports team was expected to lose, Bruce would put money on them.

I loved that he was so thoughtful. He'd get me flowers just because and leave Post-its around the house with love notes or words of encouragement.

I loved that Bruce always made sure I was comfortable and warm. Once when I was doing a photo shoot in New York, I called him during a break and mentioned that the studio was chilly. An hour later, a messenger arrived with a cashmere blanket for me and a note that said, "Stay warm." Having grown up in a single-parent household (and in itchy wool), I was shocked when I saw the price of these luxurious Frette blankets and Hermès scarves. "It's just money, Emma, and you can't take it with you," he would say, a sentiment all the more remarkable considering he was entirely self-made.

I loved that Bruce had long-standing relationships. Several friends from his struggling-actor/bartending days are still very present in our lives, and Lety, the housekeeper he hired when he started earning a bit of consistent money in his late twenties, has worked with him (and then us) for forty years.

Even though Bruce had experienced the milestones of childhood three times over with his older daughters, he embraced Mabel's and Evelyn's first words, first steps, first solid foods, and first days of school, among other moments like this, with the energy and excitement of a new father. Our girls felt seen, safe, and loved. "I'm much prouder of being a father than being an actor," he's been quoted as saying.

I loved how playful Bruce was with his daughters, especially our two young ones. If he came home and they were swimming in the pool, he'd dive in with his clothes on to get a laugh. His goal was to see our girls happy and having fun. All. The. Time. Let's just say that if he'd been solely in charge of their lives, they would have had ice cream for breakfast and probably skipped a lot of school so they could sleep in and go to the beach or Disneyland.

Bruce was also our rock during their most traumatic moments. When Mabel fell and broke her jaw the day before her sixth birthday, Bruce held her all the way to the ER and paced outside the operating room until the doctor was done. If he could have been inside supervising the surgery, he would have been. And when Evelyn slipped on the ice in our driveway and split her chin open when she was three, Bruce drove us to the hospital and cuddled her on his lap while they stitched her up. I can't count how many times he asked the doctor, "Are you sure you numbed her enough?"

I loved Bruce's authentic passion for his craft and career. It was never driven by fame or money. Okay, well maybe it was a little. He did love a payday. But mostly, it was driven by a love of acting, singing, and playing the harmonica (a skill that he proudly taught himself). The fact that he could make a living from his dream job and provide a wonderful life for his family was a bonus.

I was in awe of the aura around Bruce, one that had nothing to do with his movie star status. It's hard to put into words, but he seemed to emanate this unique magnetic energy. You could just feel it radiating off him. For example, he would walk into a restaurant or down the street with people's backs toward him and something would just make them turn around. It was wild to witness but I did, a thousand times over. When you were with Bruce, you felt you were in the presence of greatness, yet he was so simple and warm. He also had the best sense of humor. With Bruce, I was laughing from morning till night.

I loved that Bruce was a calm, sensitive, and tender Pisces. And yet, when necessary, he'd make his presence known and boundaries clear, especially when overzealous fans pushed me or the girls out of the way to get to him. Bruce didn't raise his voice, but the authority and energy he brought to those moments was something to witness. A Bruce Willis glare would send chills up your spine. His demeanor was soft, but he drew hard lines when it came to protecting his family and our time together.

I loved Bruce's strong self-confidence (where mine has always fallen short). He didn't care what others thought of him. "When you lead with integrity and good intentions, you can't let others' opinions stop you," he'd say. In less poetic moments, it was, "Fuck 'em, Emma." That's an affirmation I still use today.

When they say opposites attract, it couldn't be more spot-on than in our relationship. Bruce was a rule breaker, while I'm a rule follower. Bruce was unpredictable, while I like control, a plan, and certainty. Bruce kept me on my toes and showed me how to be nimble, to roll with life's ups and downs. (Who knew how valuable those skills would become?) He also taught me to be spontaneous, something I still try to embrace for the sake of our young girls. While I'm a worrier, Bruce didn't waste time on that. He always found joy in life. Bruce believed everyone deserved a trophy, while I'm not quite that soft and am not convinced participation alone warrants a prize. He taught me how to "live it up," as he would say, and do so to the absolute fullest. Bruce was a leader, and I was very comfortable with his take-charge personality. From watching him, I started to develop confidence of my own.

Most of all, Bruce was my protector. My parents divorced when I was seven and I would go years without seeing my father. It was traumatic to witness my mother go from a stay-at-home mom and wife to someone who had to work three jobs to support us. She always found a way to figure it out, but it was stressful to feel *her* stress and watch her navigate it alone. Probably because of this, my dream as a little girl was a picturesque life: marry Prince Charming, live in a house with a white picket fence, and have two kids. These things symbolized protection and security. And that was something Bruce gave me.

Bruce always made me feel safe when things felt hard. "Don't worry, Emma. Everything's going to be okay," he'd say when I was stressed or worried about something. Then he'd pull me close, wrap me in his arms, and kiss the top of my head. I would relax my shoulders and melt because I believed him. I could trust him. And he was usually right.

I could go on and on about the things I loved about Bruce and our life together, but what stops me in my tracks is having to use the past tense when he is alive. What a heart-wrenching gut punch. It's a quiet ache I carry daily.

WHILE THE THINGS that made me suspect Bruce was "off" started so gradually I didn't consider them symptoms, with more time, it got to the point where they were hard to ignore. I knew something was wrong. Finally, I sought medical advice, and his doctor ordered a brain scan.

Earlier, I had done a deep dive into Google, the only place I could turn for answers because of my concerns about our privacy, and found that one of the best-case scenarios would be a benign tumor pressing against his brain. My hope was that we were going to see the tumor on the scans, it would be removed, and we would go on with our lives. Unfortunately, this was not our reality. The scans showed that parts of Bruce's brain were changing, which was causing the language shifts and some of the behavior we were seeing.

In early 2022, we received a vague diagnosis of aphasia, a communication disorder that affects a person's ability to process and express language. While it was better than having no answers at all, it wasn't enough to explain the changes in Bruce's behavior. We had been in limbo for too long and the uncertainty took a toll. Chaos was building in our home, and life felt increasingly unmanageable. I realized that to get the right support for our family, I needed to understand exactly what we were dealing with.

Fast-forward to November 2022. We awaited the results of more tests. As we pulled into the parking lot of the neurologist's office, my hope was that we would leave that appointment with a clear diagnosis.

When we arrived, the nurse showed us to a room and Bruce sat on the exam table. I settled in next to him, my hand resting on his leg. After a few minutes, the neurologist walked through the door. He greeted us and made a bit of small talk. Then he said, "Bruce has primary progressive aphasia, which is a variant of frontotemporal dementia, or FTD."

From that moment on, I couldn't hear a single thing. The doctor's mouth was moving but no sound was coming out. Or maybe there was, but my ears were ringing. My hands tingled and I felt like I was free-falling.

My worst nightmare had come true.

Over the years, I'd heard horrendous stories about FTD. I'd also had doctors tell me about the various types of dementia, and when they mentioned FTD, they'd pause and say something along the lines of "Boy, that's *not* the one you want." Of course, I didn't know the full scope of it or what those letters stood for; I just knew that all types of dementias were terrible, but I had it in my head that FTD was the worst of the worst.

I had gone into that appointment thinking it would give me some relief. And while, yes, it gave me a little, there was no relief in receiving a diagnosis I didn't understand and couldn't pronounce. The only resource I was given was a flimsy pamphlet that the doctor slipped into my hand as we were ushered out of the office with a "Check back in a few months." *What? That's it?* I thought.

After that appointment, a spiral of disturbing, unsettling thoughts filled my head. Still worried about our privacy, I took another deep dive into Google. Turns out Google's a dark place to look up FTD, the most common (and some might say cruelest) form of dementia for people under the age of sixty. There is no cure or treatment; all you can do is try to manage symptoms through medication.

In that moment, I wanted nothing more than for Bruce to take charge like he used to. I wished he could pull me close, wrap his arms around me, and say, "Emma, everything's going to be okay. You worry too much." But there were no more soothing kisses on top of my head and no Bruce to help make my shoulders relax and my fear melt away. It felt like I was stepping into a new reality, uncharted terrain that I wasn't ready for.

TODAY, I AM navigating this adventure as a single parent, and it's scary. For someone who likes control and predictability, I am dealing with a disease that is anything but.

I know the details of your story are different, that your loved one is unique, that no two cases of FTD or dementia are alike. I know that no two caregiving journeys are the same either. But what I also know is that we share similar emotions watching our loved ones fade in front of our eyes, a traumatic experience that leaves a hole in your heart.

If you're picking up this book, I'm guessing it feels like your world just fell apart, too. The path of dementia is not an easy one for you, your person, or your family. But I'm here to let you know that, in time, you will find your footing. You will build confidence. You will get to the other side. You're able to handle a lot more than you think you can. Your life will take on new shape, dimension, and meaning in this next chapter, but you will find your footing and a way forward. I am telling you this because I've been there. You and I are connected by the same unfortunate, unchosen thread, but we are connected all the same.

Bruce is still a part of the fabric of my being and my guiding light, and I use the values we shared and the things he taught me to continue to make the best decisions for him and our family on his behalf and make each day the best it can be. I don't always succeed, but I try. And I do so with my biggest supporter's voice in my head: "You can do this, Emma," he tells me. "And it's going to be okay."

I want to be that supporter for you because you can do this, too, and you are not alone. We're walking this unexpected journey together.

# Making Sense of the Changing Brain

When we let go of what was and learn to
appreciate the gifts of what we have now, it will allow
us all to find joy and connection together.

**TEEPA SNOW,**
*dementia care specialist, consulting associate at*
*Duke University's School of Nursing, and founder of*
*Positive Approach to Care (PAC)*

When I suspected something was "off" with Bruce but couldn't put my finger on what it was, I went through every possible explanation in my head. Was there a problem in our marriage? Was it Bruce's sleeping difficulties?

Maybe it was his hearing loss. During the filming of the first *Die Hard* movie in the late '80s, there was a scene where he had to fire a gun underneath a table. When it was shot, oddly, Bruce wasn't wearing any protective earplugs, and he lost a large percentage of his hearing in one ear. When we first got together, this never posed a real problem.

Years later, however, I began to notice him sort of check out if we were at a dinner party or meal with the entire family. He would sit back and let everyone else do the talking without contributing very much.

Mind you, when we would get the family together, Bruce was usually the only man at a table full of women, with me, our two girls, and his three older daughters speaking a mile a minute and over each other with excitement. Initially, I thought he was just letting us have our girl time to "yack it up," as he would say, rather than trying to get a word in. I assumed his hearing loss made it easier for him to melt into his seat with his hands clasped gently on his lap.

But, in hindsight, that wasn't the Bruce I knew. Especially when it came to connecting with his daughters. Bruce was a family man at heart. Early on in our relationship and before we had children together, he wanted to spend as much time with his older girls as possible. If we were traveling, he was always dying to return home to them, calling the feeling a "gravitational pull," which always brought him back to his girls. This was something I loved about him. Today, I understand that his checking out at the table was likely due to cognitive overload and difficulty processing conversations, which is common in primary progressive aphasia (PPA), the variant of FTD that Bruce has. It was an early symptom of his disease.

## GETTING A DIAGNOSIS

Many families spend years living with a lot of confusion around symptoms prior to a diagnosis. From speaking to other care partners, I have learned how subtle (or not so subtle) symptoms of certain forms of dementia like FTD or Lewy body, for example, can rock a whole family system and destroy it. (This is not always the case with certain dementias such as Alzheimer's, where symptoms like memory issues are more obvious and usually more of a straight line to a diagnosis. Each form of dementia is different, which is why it's important not to lump them all together.)

For FTD in particular, in those early years, no one suspects the diagnosis because most people have no clue what FTD is. So they assume their person is being rude, apathetic, withdrawn, depressed, irritable, impulsive, or reckless, or they lack empathy—an array of behaviors that seem like personal choices rather than symptoms of a disease. This major shift in behavior, language, and/or personality is frustrating, confusing, and can ruin relationships. FTD is not your doctor's first or second thought either. Often FTD is misdiagnosed as a midlife crisis, depression, or bipolar disorder, to name just a few, because the symptoms can apply to all those conditions.

Bruce Miller, MD, the leading expert in FTD, distinguished professor of neurology at the University of California, San Francisco, and head of the Global Brain Health Initiative, explains:

> Many of the symptoms are very elusive and they are
> different for each neurodegenerative disease. So, while it
> may be easier to recognize that a memory problem is
> Alzheimer's, it's trickier to understand that a change in
> language or personality is FTD or another form of
> dementia. Most of us think the brain is only important for
> memory and language. But the brain is also responsible
> for our social interactions, how we relate to others, and
> how we nurture and empathize with them.

Most of us don't know this or anything else about FTD, and all you see and experience is that something is incredibly different with your loved one. Also, if you're like I was, you may feel strange bringing these things to the attention of your partner's doctor, especially if that doctor is not your own. Initially, I was uneasy going over Bruce's head in that way. Something about the morality of it didn't sit well with me. If you feel that way, too, consider the advice of Yolande Pijnenburg, PhD, a professor of young-onset dementia at Alzheimer Center Amsterdam at Amsterdam University Medical Center in the Netherlands: "If your feeling gets stronger that this change in behavior is something that person can't help, you have to trust that feeling because you're actually acting to benefit your partner."

Subtle changes due to dementia can go on for years, and all that time your person looks fine on the outside. Even more bewildering is that there might never be a moment when he or she expresses concern to you or to a doctor that something is wrong. There's actually a medical term for this: anosognosia. According to the Cleveland Clinic, anosognosia is a "condition where your brain can't recognize one or more other health conditions you have. It's extremely common with mental health conditions like schizophrenia and Alzheimer's disease. This condition isn't dangerous on its own, but people with it are much more likely to avoid or resist treatment for their other health conditions." So if your person isn't raising his or her hand for help, it's easy to think that maybe everything is okay. This makes those early stages confusing, and it's why doctors can easily overlook FTD and other early-onset dementias again and again.

"It can take at least two to three years to get a diagnosis, and in that time, many people are misdiagnosed," explains Dr. Miller. This delay can be a catastrophe, as families can be completely derailed and dismantled— emotionally and financially—by the personality changes and shifts in their loved ones from their brains quietly dying.

Over time, I began to suspect that the issue wasn't Bruce's hearing or a rocky patch in our marriage, and that instinct made me realize that we should go to the doctor. As a result of this experience, I can't stress enough the importance of trusting your gut when you know something is wrong. Even if test results come back "normal" or a doctor dismisses your concerns, don't stop pushing for answers. If your doctor isn't listening, find one who will. You know your person best. Keep advocating for them and yourself.

As I mentioned in Chapter 1, I felt some relief in finding out that Bruce had aphasia and then a year later that he had FTD. I finally understood that those crazy marital issues were not Bruce. Neither were those off moments and subtle shifts in his personality. They were the result of his brain being dismantled, taking part of the husband I knew and loved with it.

*You weren't doing any of this on purpose*, I thought as I looked over at him. *You were there the whole time.*

## WHY GETTING A DIAGNOSIS IS SO IMPORTANT

Through my experience as an FTD caregiver, I met actor Robin Williams's wife, Susan Schneider Williams, at an FTD event in San Francisco. What she told me really gets to the heart of why obtaining a diagnosis is so important:

Robin's diagnosis—Lewy body dementia (LBD)— was only made evident during an autopsy when the pathologist revealed the results and described it as one of the worst cases he'd ever seen. Though there is no cure, a diagnosis would have allowed us to seek the specialized medical care Robin needed and certain medications, which can actually speed up the disease progression, would not have been prescribed. We spent a year chasing over forty seemingly unrelated symptoms with a multitude of doctors in a diagnostic game of Whac-A-Mole. As I learned later, all of those symptoms were from the disease, which had infiltrated nearly every region of Robin's brain and brain stem. For me, knowing the diagnosis for Robin's brain disease while he was alive would have been far better.

Bruce's diagnosis was a turning point for me. Most people think that dementia is just Alzheimer's. But while it's the most common—and therefore receives all the attention—Alzheimer's is just one of many types of dementia. And not all dementias are the same. Each one progresses and affects the brain in its own way, meaning different symptoms and treatment needs.

"For example, 25 percent of people have an aphasia that doesn't develop into anything other than aphasia," dementia care specialist, consulting associate at Duke University's School of Nursing, and founder of Positive Approach to Care Teepa Snow told me. "But 75 percent develop dementia." In simple terms, for Bruce, it started with speech and spread. This is why getting the right diagnosis is so important. Each form of dementia requires different approaches to care, and understanding what you're dealing with can make all the difference in planning for the future and finding the right support.

With an actual diagnosis of FTD, I was able to get specific and tailor our next steps to Bruce's needs, which gave me a sense of control and made this journey more manageable. Having the right diagnosis also helped me plan for today and the future. It helped me grasp what FTD does, how it progresses, and what life might look like going forward. It was no longer an abstract idea or a scary, blurry outlook. Well, it was still scary, but the volume was turned down a little bit. Now I had direction.

## DIFFERENT DEMENTIAS, DIFFERENT SYMPTOMS

Many people mistakenly use the terms "dementia" and "Alzheimer's disease" interchangeably. Dementia is an umbrella term for a range of conditions that cause significant changes in multiple cognitive abilities that interfere with daily life. Alzheimer's disease is the most common type of dementia and is initially characterized by loss of immediate recall or recent memories, challenges with language processing, and other cognitive changes, primarily due to the buildup of abnormal protein plaques and tangles in the brain. It is estimated that 60 to 80 percent of dementia cases are Alzheimer's or Alzheimer's combined with another dementia. Other types of dementia include the following, courtesy of Teepa Snow:

## CHRONIC TRAUMATIC ENCEPHALOPATHY (CTE)

This type of dementia is triggered by multiple head trauma incidents over time, which cause a buildup of abnormal proteins. That accumulation results in memory loss, aggression, confusion, depression, impaired judgment, difficulty controlling impulses, erratic behavior, suicidal tendencies, anxiety, sleep disturbances, and dizziness.

## CREUTZFELDT-JAKOB DISEASE (CJD)

A rapidly progressing form of dementia caused by prion proteins, which results in sudden issues with depression, agitation, apathy, confusion, disorientation, memory, vision, hallucinations, and movement.

## FRONTOTEMPORAL DEMENTIA (FTD)

A group of disorders that cause brain cell deterioration in the frontal and temporal lobes. Depending on the specific subtype, FTD can result in personality changes, difficulty with speech production, and other cognitive issues. It can also affect movement.

## HUNTINGTON'S DISEASE

This genetic disorder causes an abnormal protein accumulation and resulting degeneration of the central area of the brain. Uncontrolled muscle movement is typically the first symptom, often followed by behavioral and personality changes and cognitive function issues.

## LEWY BODY DEMENTIA (LBD)

Lewy bodies, tiny spherical protein deposits that disrupt the function of cells throughout the brain, are seen in this form of dementia, causing symptoms such as hallucinations, delusional thinking, sleep disturbances, declined motor skills, difficulty regulating normal physical processes, and unexpected medication reactions. Memory deficits may involve more confabulation than forgetfulness, and there may be periods of typical cognition alternating with declined cognition. Lewy bodies are also present in the brains of those living with Parkinson's disease dementia.

## MIXED DEMENTIA

This involves two or more types of dementia, which scientists are realizing is much more common than previously thought.

## NORMAL PRESSURE HYDROCEPHALUS (NPH)

This type of dementia occurs due to excess cerebrospinal fluid accumulation in the brain, causing brain ventricle enlargement and damage of surrounding cells. It may result in difficulty walking, loss of bladder control, and cognitive function issues.

## POSTERIOR CORTICAL ATROPHY

This form of dementia affects the part of the brain that controls visual processing, causing challenges with reading, depth perception, movement, and other vision-related issues. Memory loss is not commonly seen until later stages of the condition. Hand-eye coordination and the ability to move safely in the world become increasingly difficult.

## PROGRESSIVE SUPRANUCLEAR PALSY (PSP)

This condition is often mistaken for Parkinson's but typically progresses more rapidly. Slow or uncoordinated movements are often the first symptoms, as well as difficulty with eye movements, loss of facial expressions, stiffness of the neck or trunk, and falls. Changes in cognitive function, behavior, and memory may also develop.

## VASCULAR DEMENTIA

This form of dementia is caused by changes in the small blood vessels of the brain, resulting in damage to the brain tissue. Hypertension, high cholesterol, diabetes, and smoking are the main risk factors for vascular dementia, which causes cognitive changes, daily fluctuations in ability, and personality and mood shifts.

## WERNICKE-KORSAKOFF SYNDROME

Triggered by a deficiency of vitamin B1 (thiamine), this form of dementia is most common in those who chronically abuse alcohol or have malabsorption. It often causes impaired memory, lack of coordination, vision issues, and personality changes.

With these wide-ranging descriptions of the various dementias, it is easy to see why it is challenging to know whether a loved one's symptoms are due to stress, environmental factors, or a condition that is going to change your entire life and the lives of everyone involved.

## RESEARCH THE DIAGNOSIS

Once you receive a diagnosis, you can begin to learn more about what is happening in the brain. A diagnosis helps identify which areas are affected, leading to changes in function. Different regions of the brain control various abilities—some involve memory, while others influence language, movement, decision-making, or emotional regulation. Understanding which areas are impacted can help you make sense of the changes in your person's behavior and responses.

For example, as Dr. Miller explains, "The frontal lobes define who we are—whether we're empathetic, whether we respect others, whether we regulate our behavior, whether we can attend properly to what other people are saying. It's our social brain and this disease attacks the social nature of us—the part of the brain that allows us to love and work with others."

This means that when the frontal lobes are affected, your person may struggle with impulse control, empathy, or emotional regulation in ways that feel unfamiliar or even hurtful. They might say inappropriate things, lose their ability to pick up on social cues, or react without considering the feelings of others. But recognizing that these changes stem from the disease—not from intent or a lack of care—can help you navigate interactions with more patience and understanding.

An accurate diagnosis also opens the potential for your loved one to participate in research trials and receive treatment that's appropriate for his or her specific condition and needs. And it helps you find the support that _you_ need. For example, you can now search for a support group with other people who are dealing with the same diagnosis you are.

"There was a twenty-three-year-old son of one of our patients in clinic who was going to an Alzheimer's support group, but all the other people were seventy, so he hated going," explains Katie Brandt, MM, director of caregiver support services in the Frontotemporal Disorders Unit at Massachusetts General Hospital, who was a caregiver for her husband before he passed away from FTD. "But then, when he found out that his dad had FTD, he found a young-onset support group. There, he connected with other guys who are in college and have a parent living with dementia and felt much less alone."

Knowledge is both powerful and empowering. In hindsight, I wish I'd read more books on dementia in the earlier stages of Bruce's disease, but I wasn't there yet. Back then, I was running around like a chicken with my head cut off. I was raising our two young girls, trying to compartmentalize and dismiss what was happening while also trying to understand it, and isolating us so I could "figure out and fix" things.

But in time, I've been able to really dig into my ongoing education. This has provided me with so much comfort and helped settle my nervous system to some degree. As Teepa says, "Knowledge is the key to stress reduction." For me, that means reading a lot and asking the doctors, specialists, and other experts about what is happening and what's to come. For you, it might mean joining a support group, whether online or in person, following dementia care experts on social media for practical tips, listening to podcasts or watching educational videos about caregiving, attending workshops or webinars on dementia care, connecting with other caregivers to share experiences and advice, keeping a journal to track changes and reflect on your emotions, or seeking professional counseling or therapy for support.

I think there's a point in the caregiving journey where you must get a little technical and methodical. Obviously, no one has a crystal ball, and doctors don't know and can't really tell me how Bruce's disease is going to progress. (Some people say, "If you've seen one person with dementia, you've seen one person with dementia.") However, they can educate me about other patients they have cared for, which helps me know what to look for and how to prepare. For example, I've learned that in the later stages of FTD, the brain's inability to coordinate certain muscles can make automatic actions like swallowing challenging and unpredictable.

When I first heard this, I was terrified. But imagine if I didn't have that information. While we're not close to that stage yet, and my hope is we never get there, it's knowledge I've stored away so I'm better equipped to care for Bruce if or when the time comes. For so long, I was paralyzed about what was happening; educating myself allowed me to stop catastrophizing and made me feel a few steps ahead. I'm a worrier and a planner—and I'm guessing a lot of you are, too. As a result, I'm all about having the information so that I'm ready as a wife, care partner, and mother, and not totally thrown when or if a change in Bruce, a new symptom, or anything else arrives at our doorstep. If it doesn't happen, then I don't need to use the knowledge I'm now armed with. But I'm glad I have it, just in case.

Having a general road map to this disease has settled my anxiety to some degree and makes me feel empowered, capable, and prepared. And that's my goal: How can I help myself feel more stable in the process? Because if I feel my feet beneath me, I'm a calmer, more effective care partner to Bruce and mother to my girls, and I'm less stressed, which is better for my own health.

Of course, if you are someone who gets overwhelmed by too much information, then just focus on what's in front of you and what you might be questioning today so you don't get too ahead of yourself. Think of three tangible items that you can tackle. It could be setting up a meeting with your neurologist, a nurse practitioner in the office, or a specialist to better understand the diagnosis and treatment plan, or creating a simple chart or calendar to track medications, appointments, and daily routines so you can avoid feeling overwhelmed. Once you're done with that, and have found your flow, add just what you need to your list. As care partners, we must do whatever we can to lower our anxiety.

## EDUCATE THOSE AROUND YOU

Have your family and friends educate themselves about your person's disease, too. And notice that I said *they* should do the educating, not *you*.

At the Association for Frontotemporal Degeneration (AFTD) 2024 Education Conference in Houston, Texas, I attended a session led by Arlene Schollaert, MSW, LCSW, and family services director of Amazing Place. She suggests getting extra pamphlets about your person's disease (like the one I was given at our diagnosis appointment) from your doctor or an advocacy organization so you can hand them out. This way, you don't need to exhaust yourself explaining the disease over and over, or fielding questions that you don't have answers to. (To this day, I have a hard time describing FTD, as there are different variants to understand, and even when I do get it right, I'm still met with a blank deer-in-the-headlights stare or the question "Does he know who you are?" Which is then followed by me saying, "Yes. He doesn't have Alzheimer's.") Let people digest the information in their own time when they are willing and want to understand more. Having family and friends learn about the disease will hopefully help get everyone on the same page about treatment (or lack of) and the everyday needs of today and what's to come. That way you're not bombarded with "Have you tried this?" or "Have you done that?" (More on this in Chapter 9.)

## FIND AN EXPERT

Prior to releasing our family's statement about Bruce's FTD diagnosis, I was too scared to talk to anyone about his condition besides his doctors. I was worried about information getting leaked before our family was ready to share it and the gossip that would ensue. But once we decided to go public, one of the first things I set out to find was a "dementia care specialist."

I wanted an expert to walk me through caring for someone with FTD and to sharpen the skills I was acquiring. Being an only child from a single-parent household, I'm a perfectionist in everything I do. Becoming a caregiver to someone I deeply love was no exception. I wanted to make sure I would do the best I could for Bruce and our family. Also, I was so desperate to connect with someone who knew the ins and outs of caregiving and could validate what I was doing correctly and tweak what I wasn't. There's an educator for everything, and I was certain there must be a dementia care specialist. I turned to Google and searched the term, and that's when Teepa Snow popped right up. I read her bio and everything about her company called Positive Approach to Care, and I thought, *She's the one.*

I reached out to make an appointment and when we spoke, Teepa was so knowledgeable about FTD, dementia, and, obviously, caregiving. She answered all my burning questions and gave me some new, fresh ideas that helped me tweak some of my caregiving skills.

It's amazing how the tiniest details can make a difference in interacting with your person and help build your confidence. For example, Teepa told me not to wear all black and suggested we replace any doormats in that color. To people with dementia, an area of black can look like a hole, so someone wearing a black T-shirt would look like they had a floating head, and a black doormat can look like a hole in the ground. She also told me to stand sideways when talking to Bruce, which is a nonconfrontational position, instead of facing him squarely, which can sometimes look aggressive to a person with dementia. Teepa was brilliant about nuances like this, and so caring. The empathy she exuded made me feel seen, heard, and less alone. Finally speaking with someone who truly understood what I was going through made me feel connected and a part of the world again.

Teepa's knowledge and guidance have been priceless for my family, but I know not everyone can afford private consultations. Thankfully, Teepa offers complimentary education on her social media pages—YouTube, Facebook, and Instagram—her website teepasnow.com, and her podcast. Her insights are accessible to anyone who needs them, making it easier for caregivers to feel supported and informed.

This is the case for many dementia and caregiving experts. You can find the right one for you by . . .

- **Exploring online resources.** Websites for organizations like the Alzheimer's Association and the Association for Frontotemporal Degeneration offer valuable information and support.

- **Connecting with a social worker or nurse in your neurologist's office.** They often have firsthand knowledge of local resources, support groups, and programs that can help guide you in the right direction.

- **Joining caregiver support groups.** You can connect with others who truly understand the journey on Facebook and in local support groups.

- **Listening to podcasts, watching YouTube videos, and following trusted experts on social media.** Try search terms such as "caregiving expert" and "dementia caregiving expert."

## UNDERSTANDING TEEPA SNOW'S FOUR TRUTHS OF DEMENTIA

One of the hardest parts of navigating dementia is coming to terms with what it really means. When Bruce was first diagnosed, I searched for anything that would give me clarity about what lay ahead. That's when I came across Teepa Snow's Four Truths of Dementia. They are difficult to hear, but they also provide an important foundation for understanding this disease:

- **At least two parts of the brain are dying.** Different forms of dementia affect different parts of the brain, impacting everything from memory and speech to personality and movement.

- **Dementia keeps changing and getting worse; it's progressive.** What works today might not work tomorrow. Symptoms evolve, and care partners must continually adapt.

- **It is not curable or fixable; it's chronic.** Unlike a temporary illness, dementia is a lifelong condition that requires ongoing management and support.

- **Dementia is terminal and results in death.** This is the hardest truth of all. It is a disease that ultimately takes the person's life.

When I first heard these truths, I remember feeling like the ground had been pulled out from under me. But over time, I realized that understanding them allowed me to shift my mindset. Instead of fighting against the inevitable, I could focus on what mattered most: making Bruce's days as meaningful and comfortable as possible, while also taking care of myself in the process.

If you're struggling with these truths, you're not alone. Let them sink in at your own pace and know that while you can't change the reality of dementia, you *can* change how you approach it.

## SEPARATE THE PERSON FROM THE DISEASE

Teepa's book *Understanding the Changing Brain: A Positive Approach to Dementia Care* became an important read for me. Not only was I able to understand the workings of a healthy brain, I understood what happens to a person's brain when they have dementia. A closer look at how Bruce's brain was changing didn't make it any less devastating; this whole experience was and will always be heartbreaking to me.

However, when I realized that Bruce's brain was changing, it allowed me to separate him from his disease. That was big. I still have anger and resentment, but it is not directed at Bruce; it is directed at the disease of FTD, and I'm still pissed at it. There is a big difference, and I hope and encourage you to use this insight to reframe your thinking, too. When I started to understand Bruce's limitations, which were no fault of his own but the result of his changing brain, it truly transformed my outlook and experience as a care partner.

As Teepa explains:

> At first, you think the individual knows what he's doing when he says or does things he's never done before. Or you think that he understands you. But he has actually been robbed of these abilities by the dementia. It's like a thief that comes in and steals away that piece of the brain. A person living with dementia is doing the best he or she can at any given moment. It's up to us to recognize this and try to figure out how to support them so we can all thrive together.

Teepa also taught me to tell myself, *What he's saying or doing is not a choice. It's what's left of his brain.* That's when you realize that this behavior isn't the person you love. It's the dementia *within* the person you love.

"They're built into the same person," Teepa told me. "So, it's super important to realize the difference between the individual and the dementia. Otherwise, if you hate their dementia, it gets easy to believe that you hate them, too. And you don't. You love them. You're just so frustrated with their dementia."

FRANCIS BACON FAMOUSLY said, "Knowledge is power." This holds true in many aspects of life, but especially as a care partner. For me, the more I learned about the brain and Bruce's condition, the better equipped I felt to manage my responsibilities, like balancing caregiving with the demands of our family's daily life and planning for what lay ahead. Gaining a deeper understanding of FTD not only shaped how I approached each day and the care Bruce received, but it also eased my nervous system, giving me a sense of calm and control, however small. Most importantly, it allowed me to better understand the person I love most, my husband, so I could care for him with greater compassion and intention.

The same can be true for you. The more you understand your loved one's condition, the more empowered you'll feel to navigate the road ahead. Knowledge won't change the reality of the disease, but it can change how you show up, how you cope, and how you find moments of peace within the uncertainty.

## QUESTIONS AND ANSWERS
## WITH TEEPA SNOW

I can't tell my story of caring for Bruce without talking about Teepa and how much support and clarity she provided for me, our family, and eventually our formal caregivers. Here is more of her priceless insight.

**Why is it important for you to teach people how to understand the changing brain?**

Understanding the basics of how the brain works will help us become more aware that, with dementia, there are changes that cannot be reversed; but at the same time, there are abilities we can maximize to make life more satisfying for all. Also, we've asked families to care for individuals with zero training. Nothing. You don't get anything from the doctor, and you get nothing from a specialist. You're basically told, "Do the best you can, and after that I have some meds that might help—but they might not—and they're not going to change the disease. Oh, and you'll probably need to put the individual someplace eventually." In other words, you're being told that this disease will get worse and then it'll get *a lot* worse. And then you hear that your days are going to now be thirty-six hours long, there's nothing good about it, it's going to be awful, and it'll tear you apart. What a horrible way to go into the next five to eight to ten to twelve to fifteen years of your life. But if you understand the changes happening in the brain, then you can start to build changes into your life. You can figure out how to adapt. Because it's not all horrible and awful. Yes, it's hard and I wouldn't wish it on my worst enemy. But if it happens, it happens. So how do you live through it and learn from it? How do you build a new life because that's all you can do? And how do you come to terms with this and move forward? Otherwise, you're just wasting time wanting what you can't have.

### Why is it important to get a diagnosis and know the difference between each type of dementia?

The more we know with a specific diagnosis, the better position we can put ourselves in to succeed. I find it totally unhelpful to keep labeling something as Alzheimer's that is not. Why? Because each form of dementia is very different, so depending on the diagnosis, the individual's abilities will be very different. People think, What does it matter? Especially because there are not special drugs for each condition. But a clear diagnosis is about living life. You can do this so much more wisely with the right supports in place and with training on that specific disease. For example, when I was working with you and Bruce, it was clear that words were challenging for him. So I told you and the people around him to quit using so many words or it would tick him off. Instead, it was more helpful to use simple gestures.

Knowledge is the key to stress reduction. Learn about the changes that happen when someone develops dementia and how this might impact expectations, interactions, interests, relationships, and outcomes. Then you can put the right support in place—support for you, support for the individual, support for the family, and support for your finances, as well.

**Is it correct to say that the brain is dying, or is it misfunctioning?**

Early in the condition, the brain experiences some dysfunction. Changes in the brain cells and the chemicals that transmit messages between cells can cause some misfiring. But by the time we're saying the word "dementia," it means there's tissue that's dying and is no longer available. Other tissue that's left in the brain steps up to the plate and says, "I'll help," which is where you get forbidden words coming out of the individual's mouth, or they are doing things they would never have done before. It's typically control over impulses, decision-making, sequencing, language, and comprehension that are impacted.

*Something to think about . . .*

What additional information can you seek out about your loved one's disease and where can you find that information?

_____

_____

_____

_____

_____

_____

_____

_____

# THREE

# Build Community and Connection

There is no sidestepping the grief, the
pain, the helplessness. There is just, maybe,
a human wall of comfort to lean on.

**PATTI DAVIS,**
*in her* New York Times *op-ed "Bruce Willis,*
*My Father and the Decision of a Lifetime"*

At my daughter Mabel's sixth-grade graduation, each child had to get up and give a short speech. One of Mabel's classmates talked about the importance of community, and he started with this definition, which I thought was beautiful: "Community: noun, a feeling of fellowship with others as a result of sharing common attitudes, interests, and goals." I was struck by this because I know that leaning into the caregiving community was vital for me in making sense of this journey; it was the game changer I didn't know I needed. And for a long time, I resisted it.

I told myself I could handle it alone, that asking for help was unnecessary or even a sign of failure. But the truth is, what I have learned is that no one can do this alone and we shouldn't have to. If we are to make it through this journey without completely losing ourselves, we have to allow others in. We have to reach out, even when it feels uncomfortable, because caregiving is not meant to be done in isolation. In fact, that can be dangerous.

From a very young age, one thing I internalized from my parents' divorce was that you should probably never depend on anyone but yourself. Overnight, we went from a middle-class family to one where my mom and I were struggling to stay afloat. But my mom rose to the occasion. As a single parent, she did whatever she needed to do to make sure there was food on our table, a roof over our heads, and gifts under the Christmas tree. Nothing was beneath her, whether it was cleaning people's homes or handing out food samples at the grocery store. Eventually, she became an agent to actors at a small agency in Orange County, California, a modeling agent when we moved back to London, the creator of her own fashion magazine, and then my manager when I started to model. Her hustle was real and relentless, and she did it all by herself. As a result, she raised me to be independent and make my own way in the world so I would never need to rely or depend on anyone. But what I also learned was to bottle up my feelings, put on a brave face, and push through. To me, asking for help meant you were not self-sufficient, and perhaps even weak.

We all have our trauma that we carry with us. When I look back on mine, I know it's what has made me who I am today—strong, resourceful, and resilient. I'm grateful for the life lessons I've gained and how much they have helped me walk through this new chapter of my life knowing that I can take it on at any stage as a single parent. Watching my mom taught me that we can do hard things on our own, and we don't always need to ask for help. But I'm learning to untangle that web because it does *not* apply to being a care partner. There is just no way you can do this without help. (And it's not just me saying that. Every expert and care partner I've spoken to for this book and on this journey with Bruce has said the same thing. Every. Single. One.)

When I suspected something was going on with Bruce but didn't have an answer, asking for help never even crossed my mind. Instead, I remained extremely isolated trying to understand and manage what was happening on my own. I also kept these suspicions to myself because, as I mentioned earlier, I worried about gossip and fodder for the tabloids. *Who could I trust?* I thought. *And what would I say anyway?* I was young with young kids and a youngish husband, so even if I had wanted to find my people, I didn't know anyone who could relate to my situation. I had so little information that I didn't even know what kind of support we'd need, if any. Also, as Bruce's disease progressed, I was raising two small kids, so the number of adult conversations I was having on a daily basis dwindled rapidly. I felt like the world was closing in on me.

Can you relate to this feeling of wanting to isolate? Manage everything yourself? Not reach out to anyone? Maybe it's because, like me, you were raised to be strong and handle things on your own, and you think no one else can understand. Or you have this idea that caregiving for a member of your family should only be done by you. Perhaps you think it's weak to ask for help, or you don't want to burden others. But no one can travel this road alone.

All caregiving journeys can feel lonely and isolating, but the dementia caregiver's path often feels even more so. The absence of shared decision-making or meaningful conversations with your loved one amplifies that sense of isolation. Because Bruce can't communicate with me (due to the variant of FTD he has, primary progressive aphasia), I must make judgment calls for him about absolutely everything. I can't ask him how he's feeling, what's wrong, or if something hurts. Instead, I read his body language or look into his eyes to understand what's bothering him and what he's experiencing. I compare this to the instinct that you have as a parent. With just one glance at your child, you can tell immediately if something isn't right. And with one look at Bruce, I can tell if his neck hurts or if he's got a headache. This responsibility puts added stress on the caregiver. Without you, your person can't care for themselves, so not only are you dealing with your feelings, your person's life is literally in your hands. It's no wonder caregivers put themselves on the back burner time and time again. We are so laser-focused on our person.

Ultimately, to take care of your loved one, you need to take care of *you*. This means having a safe space to reveal your thoughts and vent openly, cry, or laugh. A safe space to learn tips and tricks, find resources, receive feedback on areas that might use some improvement, and get some validation. That safe space is your caregiver community.

"We do not yet have a cure for dementia, but *we do* have a cure for the isolation and loneliness that may come with a diagnosis," says Katie Brandt of the Frontotemporal Disorders Unit at Massachusetts General Hospital. "That cure is your community."

## WHY COMMUNITY MATTERS

When you are part of a community and in the presence of people who understand what you're going through, you can exhale. Community is not having to walk in with your chest pumped up. You can let your shoulders slump. You can melt into all your feelings. You don't have to put on a show. You can truly be yourself.

Bruce always used to tell me, "Chin up. Chest out." This works when I'm out in the world and talking to people in general, especially when I'm asked the very complicated question "How's Bruce doing?" I really don't know how to answer that. My triggered, unhinged response would be "Well, he has FTD. *How do you think he's doing?!*" Yes, I know when people ask that, it is coming from a place of concern and love. And of course, it's better they ask than skirt by it; I just have a hard time responding without spiraling. But when I'm with my people, my community, my shoulders relax, I can cry, and no one is confused or wondering what's going on. I can just be me, my rawest, most true authentic self. And come to think of it, those in my community don't even ask me how Bruce is doing, because they know how complicated it is to answer that question. Instead, they say, "How are you and the girls holding up?" They get me. They understand me. They validate me. And on this uncertain path, that kind of support and to feel seen are priceless.

Also, when you're with your community, you're not being judged. As I mentioned earlier, it sometimes feels as if the only emotion we are allowed to express as caregivers is sadness. Sharing any others, like frustration, grief, anger, resentment, exhaustion, or even moments of joy, can lead to a lot of judgment from those who are not care partners because, in their eyes, the person we are caring for has it worse than we do. There is no question we understand that dementia is happening *to* our loved ones, and trust us, if we could take this disease away from them and claim our lives back, we'd do it in a heartbeat. Still, we experience a range of feelings and complicated emotions, and we should be able to express them without judgment. Because if you can't be real with family and friends and instead feel misunderstood, you will end up isolating, and isolation is bad for both your physical and mental health. You need to be able to express yourself and have meaningful conversations or else you're going to bubble over. They don't call it dis-ease for nothing. (Some holistic doctors hyphenate "dis-ease" to emphasize the idea that illness [dis] stems from an imbalance or disruption in overall well-being [ease], whether physical, emotional, or spiritual.)

"Caregivers' feelings are complex. Of course, there's love," explains Habib Sadeghi, DO, cofounder of Entelechy Medical Center, an integrative health center based in Los Angeles, whom I have the privilege of speaking with twice a month about my personal situation. "But if you don't acknowledge the guilt, shame, grief, and loss, you cannot access the love, and if you stay with the guilt, shame, grief, and loss, it wears on you and this is a recipe for addiction, anxiety, burnout, and confusion." Your community is a good place to find others experiencing similar emotions. In fact, your health and sanity depend on it.

Look, I get it. No one *wants* to be a part of this community, because when you are, it means that your person is sick. No one signs up for it. But since you aren't given the luxury of a choice, I encourage you to lean into it, allow yourself to be embraced by it, and find the support you need. Ask for help, accept the help, and take advantage of all that people on this journey have to offer. Community and connection are beautiful parts of this journey; these are very meaningful layers in my life, and the sooner you become a part of it, the better.

I now have a small inner circle of people who have walked this road before me. They inspire me and provide me with so much comfort, and I learn from them daily. One of the best things about finally finding my people was realizing that everyone shares the same feelings, even though our stories may be different. When you're a caregiver to someone who has dementia, all those feelings are one parcel. But you don't know that until you talk to others who are going through it, too. Trust me, the relief you will feel when you realize this and the deep exhale you'll be able to take are like nothing else.

There are several types of people who have helped me most on my journey. I'll share them in the following sections, in hopes that they can guide you in finding your people, too.

## THE PERSON WHO'S AHEAD OF YOU ON THE JOURNEY

One of the most important members of your community is the person who's walking a few steps ahead of you on the caregiving journey, because they can provide insight but aren't so removed that they can't empathize with what you're currently going through. For me, that person is my friend Franne.

Holding it together during the process of seeking a diagnosis for Bruce wasn't easy. As you can imagine, this was a confusing and stressful time, and I was still keeping things quiet. One of the few people in my inner circle was another of Bruce's closest friends, songwriter, record producer, and studio executive Robert Kraft. Robert and Bruce have known each other for decades, prior to Bruce becoming famous. In fact, when Bruce flew out to Los Angeles to audition for *Moonlighting*, he crashed on Robert's couch. All to say, Robert knows Bruce as well as anyone and had noticed something was off, too. He also saw how the stress of this confusing situation was affecting me. One night, he called me.

"I have someone for you to speak to who is going through a very similar thing," Robert said. "Her name is Franne Golde. She's an amazing songwriter and close friend whom I've worked with for decades, and her husband, Paul, has young-onset Alzheimer's. I know she's someone you can trust." Paul, who was around Bruce's age, was in the prime of his life, as was Franne, when Paul was diagnosed.

At first, I was skeptical. *How could anyone grasp the true complexity of my reality?* I wondered. Yes, Franne and I shared the common thread of having a spouse living with cognitive changes, and the ensuing grief. However, Franne's husband had a clear diagnosis, and at the time, we did not. In fact, never in my wildest dreams did I think Bruce had a form of dementia. Also, at this point, the real intense sadness had not set in yet. I was still in denial that I had a husband who wasn't well; I wasn't talking freely about this to anyone, even my mother, whom I tell everything to. I was also in cover-up mode and didn't realize how much this was weighing on me, so I was unsure how connecting with someone else would really help.

Luckily, despite my hesitation, Robert pushed me to reach out to Franne. I was so used to putting smoke and mirrors in place to protect Bruce and our family that before the first call, I had to tell myself, *Emma, be honest. Be truthful.* I guess I listened to my own advice because my friendship with Franne was formed from the word "hello." The second we started talking, I couldn't stop sharing. Although her husband had a diagnosis and Bruce didn't, our stories and feelings were so similar. I was able to put it all out there: my initial worry that my marriage was failing, concern that I didn't have a language for what was happening, and the discomfort and uncertainty I felt about having a husband facing illness. Franne could relate, and she listened and validated what I had been experiencing. When she said, "I totally get it, Emma," it was such a relief. The balloon of shame, grief, sadness, and resentment that I had been carrying instantly deflated. These were emotions I didn't realize I was experiencing until I expressed them. Tears filled my eyes, and I felt like I was home.

I think you will feel the same relief when you open up to someone who's on this journey, because when they say, "I get it" or "Me too," it can feel like someone has taken that one-hundred-pound backpack off your shoulders. There's that saying "We are only as sick as our secrets," and I think it's true. Finding someone you are comfortable and confident talking to is freeing, and you want to be as free as possible on this journey. Unburdening yourself in this way is one of the few things you can control in a situation that is mostly out of your control.

Franne and I have been talking and building a close friendship ever since. She holds no judgment, and I can trust her with all my emotions. Sometimes I call her just to have a good old messy cry. When I tell her what I'm feeling, she understands because she's experienced it all, too. There are things I can talk to Franne about that no one else would understand, and things we can laugh about that no one else would find funny. (Finding humor in this journey is important!) I am in awe of her strength and grateful to have her a few steps ahead of me. Our connection has also taught me to be more honest and to trust that I can bring people into the fold to listen and maybe even help rather than remain guarded and build walls.

One day Franne told me how they revealed Paul's diagnosis to their family, friends, and colleagues in a Facebook post.

"It was just so freeing," she explained. At the time, I was doing all I could to hide my suspicion that something was wrong with Bruce, so I envied her ability to be so open. *To be able to live in your truth? What a relief! That must be so liberating*, I thought. The ability to be that honest was my goal. Eventually, when our family shared the news of Bruce's diagnosis with the public, it was partly because Franne had served as an example of the relief this kind of honesty could bring. With her help, I realized I don't have to mask my emotions all the time and keep going, and that there's no need to distance myself from everything and everyone. If I continued to do that, I would only deepen the sense of isolation I was already drowning in.

In December 2022, Franne lost her beloved Paul to complications from young-onset dementia. Witnessing her unwavering love and the tenderness with which she cared for Paul deeply shaped my own path as a care partner.

---

"You want to have people around you who say, 'I know it's hard, but there is hope. I want you to know that greater is coming. I want you to know that you will have the ability to smile again. I want you to know that weeping may endure for a night, but joy will come in the morning.' But it's only other caregivers who can say this because they understand your grief and the need to find hope."

**TY LEWIS,**
*advocate, educator, and certified dementia*
*practitioner who is her mother's caregiver*

---

## THE PERSON WHO CAN GIVE YOU
## HONEST FEEDBACK

Another benefit to having someone in your corner who knows what you're going through is that they can look out for you like few others can. Sometimes this means offering tough love or a dose of the truth when you need it. For me, that person was also Franne. Before we got the FTD diagnosis for Bruce, we were invited on a trip to Mexico. It was going to be me, Bruce, Mabel and Evelyn, our close family friends, and someone to help me support Bruce. My gut told me that this might be the last family trip we would be able to share with him. Although taking someone with cognitive challenges out of their environment and routine can be difficult, his neurologist had given me a cautious green light, understanding how much this trip meant to me. I'd carefully dotted every i and crossed every t to make it safe and comfortable for Bruce to go, and Mabel and Evelyn were very excited to have this time together. We were a week away from traveling when I told Franne about going to Mexico.

"Emma. What are you doing?" she said. "Don't take him out of his routine. It's not going to be any kind of break for you and it's not going to be the trip you envision or one that you'll want to remember. You can't do it." My stomach sank and my heart broke, even though I knew she was right. Franne had walked in my shoes, so I heard what she was telling me loud and clear. I wasn't happy about it, but I had to listen. *Okay, I'll cancel our trip*, I thought while she was talking.

"But don't cancel *your* trip," she went on. "You're still going with the kids. They're looking forward to it, you need it, and they should see you having fun and not just stressed all the time. And you know Bruce would want you and the kids to go."

I listened to her, and the girls, our friends, and I went to Mexico. And boy oh boy, did I have guilt and shame around that decision. On top of this, our girls initially were upset their dad wouldn't be joining us. But when I explained why, they got it. Even at their young ages, they knew what the day-to-day looked like with Bruce because they were very much a part of it. They understood the level of care that he would need; this wouldn't just magically disappear because we were in Mexico. In fact, we'd need even more thoughtfulness and attention.

Taking our first family trip without Bruce was crushing, but Franne was right, and I appreciated her honesty. It wouldn't have been the magical trip I was envisioning. It would have been like being at home, only somewhere else, and therefore more stressful for everyone, including Bruce. I was able to put the right care into place back home for Bruce and we wound up having a beautiful time. Of course, I still worried about him every day, but I made sure to not amplify it more than necessary. It was so healthy for the girls to see me completely removed from caregiving and just being their mom. The fact that we could nonchalantly run, splash, and play in the ocean without thinking and worrying about every detail was a luxury and the respite the girls and I needed.

Franne was my first link to community, and I am beyond grateful for her and to Robert for introducing us. So how can you find your Franne, someone who is a few steps ahead of you on the journey and can give you feedback, even when it's hard to hear? First, get clear on what you're looking for. Then, if you're open to it, manifest it.

Now, let me start by saying I'm a very practical thinker. I'm not really into anything woo-woo. If I don't see it and I can't touch it, it's hard for me to believe it. But what I've learned on this journey is sometimes the road of dementia can get so difficult that we just have to trust the process and believe that there is something bigger than ourselves—which can be your God, Lord, Mother of all creations, or even something intangible that you don't have a name for—that can guide us and bring things forward to us. I wouldn't say I believed in manifesting or even fully understood the concept at first. But looking back, there have been moments in my life when I manifested exactly what I needed, simply because I was so clear and grounded in what I was seeking.

In fact, I think I manifested Bruce. After my ex-fiancé and I broke up, I was having lunch with a friend when she asked me what my next ideal partner would look like. "A man who has a job and a sense of humor, who is warm, fun, and kind," I told her. That's Bruce in a nutshell, and four weeks later, he reappeared in my life.

Whether you call it manifesting or not, I believe that our thoughts are powerful, both positively and negatively, so we have to be conscious of them. If this resonates with you, why not put it out into the universe that you're looking for your Franne? Say out loud or write down what you are looking for: "I'm trying to find someone who is ___ and ___." Even if this seems a bit out there, it can't hurt. Just be clear and specific and see what happens.

Also, tap into your network. Ask your neurologist's office if they know another family in a similar situation wanting to make a connection. Tell friends what you're looking for. Ask the pastor of your church, the rabbi of your temple, or any other community leader if they know someone who has a loved one with dementia and if they can introduce you. If you're comfortable with social media, post to Facebook or Instagram. In my experience, there are many people on social media looking to connect on this subject. Just note that your Franne doesn't have to be that far ahead of you in the journey for you to find support, connection, and a safe haven.

## THE PERSON WHO IS YOUR ROLE MODEL

Another important person to have in your community is a role model, or someone you can look up to as an example of navigating this journey. For me, that person is Patti Davis, an author and the daughter of President Ronald Reagan. In 2004, he passed away from complications from Alzheimer's at the age of ninety-three. Patti is a friend and mentor, and I wouldn't know her if not for the fact we've both had loved ones with dementia. Let me explain how we met.

In early 2023, a few weeks after we released our family statement about Bruce's FTD diagnosis, someone sent me an op-ed piece Patti had written for *The New York Times* called "Bruce Willis, My Father and the Decision of a Lifetime." She wrote that our story reminded her of when her father shared his diagnosis with the country five years after he left the White House. "My fellow Americans," President Reagan wrote, "I have recently been told that I am one of the millions of Americans who will be afflicted with Alzheimer's disease." Patti talked about how her mother, Nancy Reagan, called her a few hours before the letter was released to the public. Patti understood the complexities of sharing this information with the world.

After that call, she went on a walk, to have those last few hours of privacy before the news about her father went public. Without knowing,

I had done the exact same thing. I took a walk the evening before our statement went out, prayed, had a good cry, and just said, "Fuck it." I didn't know what was going to happen with the public and the media, but it really didn't matter. Sharing the news was about saving our family, putting everything into place with no more smoke and mirrors. We would embrace this new chapter of our lives, be transparent, and live our full truth. This would also help our young daughters. I never wanted them to think that their dad's diagnosis was a family secret they had to keep. I didn't want them to ask about their father's disease in hushed tones. There is nothing to be ashamed of. This was not his fault. I didn't want any kind of stigma attached to his diagnosis. It also was important for our girls to see our family go out and raise awareness on a global scale, because that is the kind of reach that their father has. And I wasn't going to let FTD write our family's story; we would. I knew Bruce would want our family to do whatever we needed to do to bring peace into our lives while being able to help others.

In that op-ed, Patti wrote:

> My hope for Bruce Willis's family, as they go down this unpredictable and heartbreaking road, is for those around them to know that simply being there is often all you can do. There is no sidestepping the grief, the pain, the helplessness. There is just, maybe, a human wall of comfort to lean on.
>
> I experienced that, I felt it—the concern and compassion of strangers who took time out of their lives to think about us, to care about how we were doing. And there are others

whom the Willis family will never meet, other families who have been invaded by this cruel disease, who today feel a little less lonely because of the decision to announce a diagnosis that rips your soul apart.

When I read those words, I felt an instant connection to Patti, even though I didn't know her. I appreciated her thoughtfulness and that she understood the vast difference between an Alzheimer's diagnosis and an FTD one. She saw the whole complicated picture, which made me feel seen. I thought about picking up the phone to call her, but I didn't have her number. Also, I was in the process of learning and understanding how to lean into and on this community. To be honest, I was in disbelief that I needed to be a part of it. *I'm young, and so is my husband*, I thought.

Time went on and then one day, I got a text from Maria Shriver, a longtime family friend and mentor, who said, "I have a book for you that Patti Davis would like me to drop off." My heart skipped a beat. The book was *Floating in the Deep End: How Caregivers Can See Beyond Alzheimer's*. I loved everything about that book. I loved how open and raw Patti was, with no BS on any subject. Reading it, I felt validated. I underlined page after page. I still keep it close by to reference. Inside the book was a simple handwritten card from Patti with her phone number that said, "Call me if you ever need me." She didn't have to ask me twice. I called straightaway! And I'm happy to say we've been friends ever since.

Patti taught me a lot about the importance of community and connection, and I so appreciate her incredible, no-nonsense insight. She has given so much back to the caregiving community by sharing her story, writing her books, and starting support groups. You'll hear more from Patti later in this chapter and book, but having her as a role model, someone much further along in the journey than me, has been instrumental. Try to seek out that person in your life because their wisdom and the lessons they'll teach you are invaluable. You don't even have to meet that person to view them as a role model. In fact, even if I hadn't met Patti, her book taught me so much and put her in that position in my life.

Here are some ways you can tap into your role model's wisdom without ever meeting them:

- **Read their books.** Many experts share their knowledge through memoirs, guides, and research-based books.

- **Listen to their podcasts.** Hearing their voice and perspective can offer reassurance and practical advice.

- **Watch their talks or interviews.** Many thought leaders speak at conferences or summits, or share insights via YouTube.

- **Follow their social media or blogs.** Many caregivers and experts regularly post advice, reflections, and community support.

- **Attend virtual or in-person conferences and support groups.** Learning from those who have been through it can be incredibly valuable. Even if you never meet them in person, these role models can still provide guidance, strength, and a sense of solidarity.

"Caregivers need to talk to each other.
Human contact is so helpful when you're caring
for someone with dementia. You cannot do this
walk alone. Finding other people can get us
through a lot of hard times."

**PAULINE BOSS,**
*PhD, professor emeritus at the University of Minnesota
and author of six books, including* Loving Someone Who Has
Dementia, *who was a caregiver for her husband*

## A SUPPORT GROUP

There is strength, understanding, and insight in the caregiving community. There is hope, too. And you can find all that through a support group. But the biggest benefits come from realizing that your experience and the emotions that go with it are shared by others. You are not alone.

"You may think, *Nobody will understand this. Nobody else feels like this,* and then you'll see that you're sitting with ten to fifteen or more people, and they all get what you're talking about," explains Patti. They've thought and felt the same things but also felt like they were alone.

Patti told me that in the groups she ran, there were plenty of times when someone would say, "Sometimes I can't wait for this to be over." And guess what? Not one person was shocked, confused, or told them, "How can you say that?" That's the beauty of a shared experience.

"You're a human being, and you're allowed to have those thoughts. In a support group, you can express them," Patti said.

Another benefit of participating in a support group is being surrounded by people who are at different parts of the journey than you are. Some are just starting, some are in the middle, and some may even be done. You can help those who are steps behind you, and it's an incredible feeling to support others the way you wish you had been supported and to gain insight from those who are a little ahead of you. You can also find hope when you hear from caregivers who have made it to the other side and are okay. What a beautiful realization in a situation that can be so scary and uncertain. Plus, chances are any issue or problem you're having, someone else in the group has experienced it and can offer insight and comfort.

There is also something nice about the accountability of a group that meets regularly. Not only can you brainstorm ideas together, but the group gets to know you and how your journey is progressing. It's also, as we learned earlier, a place you may find your Franne. And even if you don't, that's okay; you can still find people to laugh with.

"People with dementia do and say funny things but only other caregivers will understand the humor," says Patti, who told me that they laughed a lot in the groups she ran.

One way to find a support group that's right for you is to reach out to organizations that focus on your person's disease, such as the Association for Frontotemporal Degeneration (AFTD) or the Alzheimer's Association, which also covers other forms of dementia. (More suggestions on my website, emmahemingwillis.com.) Today, thanks to how comfortable we've gotten being virtual, there are several online support groups for caregivers. You can also join one on Facebook or another social media platform or start your own by posting something about how you're creating a support group and then being specific about what type of group it is.

Just one sidenote: It may take some trial and error to find the right support group for you, so don't be discouraged if you don't feel a connection with the first group you try. I'd suggest going a few times, and if it just doesn't feel right, try another group.

---

"Connecting with others in similar situations is incredibly powerful and lessens the sense of being alone. Sharing one's story with others is so meaningful, healing, and can offer optimism and hope on a very difficult path."

**DAVID PFEIFER,**
*who was a care partner to his wife who had FTD*

---

## AN ORGANIZATION

Another important part of your community can be an organization centered around your loved one's disease. For me, AFTD is where I've been able to find resources and connect with other care partners. Just one month after releasing our family's second statement about Bruce's FTD diagnosis, I attended my first ever FTD event, the AFTD Hope Rising Benefit in New York, where I was surrounded by caregivers past and present. I could see the wounds and trauma so deeply embedded in them, and their touch and nods of understanding were warm, reassuring, and hopeful. They had a special look in their eyes. When you meet someone who has walked in your shoes and experienced how devasting this disease is, the playing field is leveled, even when your husband is Bruce Willis. At that event, I felt seen, maybe for the first time in my life.

As you build out your community, find the association for your loved one's specific type of dementia and visit their website. They offer a lot of information and an array of resources such as support groups, helplines, caregiver support days and events, grants for respite care, research studies, and opportunities to give back, among others.

## PLACES TO FIND YOUR COMMUNITY

- At your neurologist's office—ask if there is another family or caregiver they can put you in touch with

- Your church, temple, or other place of worship

- Social media groups

- Your local hospital

- Organizations like AFTD or the Alzheimer's Association

- Word of mouth—tell friends and family members you're looking for another dementia caregiver to connect with

- Adult day health programs near you

- A local memory care center

- Start your own support group. You can do this by posting on social media or—the old-fashioned way—by hanging a sign on a local bulletin board.

## YOUR FRIENDS WHO ARE NOT CAREGIVERS—WHEN YOU'RE READY

It's hard to vent, cry, complain, and even laugh with people who don't understand what it means to be a care partner. Even if you have extended family members or close friends who visit your person often, unless they are living with you and your loved one every moment, they'll never grasp how hard it is, how traumatic it is, and how sad it is to have that front-row seat to your person's disease as it slowly progresses day-to-day. So while your friends who are not caregivers can also be an important part of your community, bringing them into the fold may take some time.

In the beginning, I had no desire to go out and connect with people who weren't on this journey. I had been diagnosed with depression, so having to put on a brave and happy face or act as if nothing was happening was too exhausting to even think about. I also didn't want to have to explain myself and was too fragile to answer a lot of probing questions and educate someone on the disease. For example, the worst questions I would get from people who didn't know the dementia experience were (and still are) "How's Bruce feeling? Is he better?" Those questions are triggering and exhausting because I have to explain that you don't get better from this disease. There's no cure or treatment. It's a horrible thing to discuss and hear myself say out loud.

So I avoided plans. I said no to invitations more than I said yes, and I was closed off. Eventually, and yet not surprisingly, those invitations stopped coming and those friendships or potential friendships left the station. Honestly, at the time I was too drained and shell-shocked to even care. But I had made the mistake of not being honest with my friends about why I was declining invite after invite. Don't do that. Instead, let your friends know why you are saying no. They will appreciate this honesty and know not to take it personally. Then tell them to try again in a month.

It's only more recently that I will meet up with a friend who does not have this shared experience. Part of why I'm now able to do so is that Bruce is more settled in his disease (as am I with his diagnosis), and I have the right support in place. The other reason is knowing that one of the pillars of brain health is social connection (more on this in Chapter 5). I need to be in the real world, not just for my health, but also to be a role model for my kids. I don't want them to see me not going out, having friends, or seeking joy.

I started by having coffee or lunch with those I considered safe people, those who wouldn't ask questions that would trigger me and to whom I could comfortably say, "I don't want to talk about this anymore." I'm grateful to have a handful of these supportive friends who know how to read the room, and I trust them immensely.

The truth is, it's great to have community in *both* worlds, but getting there can take a while. When you are ready, I suggest you spend time with these non-caregiver friends, too. There *is* something nice about being able to disconnect from this one-note topic of living with dementia, day in and day out, so you can feel "normal." (Gosh, normal? What does that even feel like?)

But in all fairness, you have to be ready to reengage with that second world because it does take a high level of strength and energy. When you do meet up with these friends, it's okay to set an expectation from the beginning. For example, you can say that you don't want to talk about your person or caregiving because you need a true break from it all. Or that you'll limit your update to the first five minutes but then want to move on. Most people will understand and respect your boundaries.

## SOMEONE WHO CAN USE YOUR WISDOM

Part of belonging to the caregiving community is the ability to be there for someone else, whether you're a few steps ahead of them on the journey, are their role model or a member of their support group, or are just someone who can connect them with resources or lend a listening ear. Recently, I met a woman whose loved one was newly diagnosed with FTD-ALS. (This is where symptoms of both disorders—frontotemporal dementia and amyotrophic lateral sclerosis, also known as Lou Gehrig's disease—are present.) She asked for help. Connecting her to the right information and resources was a moment I won't forget. Even though I couldn't change her situation, I could guide her, tell her where to start, and make her feel a little less lonely. I could be that someone in her corner who understands her experience and offers her some hope. Giving back in this small way not only strengthens my sense of community but is part of reframing this journey. I can't help the fact that I'm on it, but I can turn it into something positive. (Read more about reframing this journey in Chapter 10.)

WHEN WE RELEASED our first statement about Bruce's health and the fact that he was stepping away from his career in March of 2022, I was nervous, especially because we didn't have a final diagnosis. What we had was a symptom of a disease, aphasia.

Even without a diagnosis, being able to come out to the public was a blessing. In the months that followed, there was a huge outpouring of compassion. Many people reached out with messages of concern and support because Bruce is so beloved. I was fortunate enough to stand below to catch that waterfall of kindness they showered on him.

The doom, gloom, and immense sadness of this disease will always be there. I'm always waiting for the next shoe to drop. When I see a change or decline in Bruce, I go into a tailspin for a few weeks. This involves a lot of crying, worrying, what-if thinking, catastrophizing, being short-fused with everyone around me, anger, sadness, and grief. I am totally unbalanced and out of whack. All I want to do is isolate, but what I know now is *that* is when I must lean on my community and reach out. Because I am no longer alone. I'm part of a community.

You cannot do this by yourself. Hope on the caregiving journey lies in finding other people. That is what can get us through the worst of times. Yes, we come from all walks of life, but our stories and experiences with the disease are common ground. This is so powerful, and I find solace in that. In community, you feel seen and heard. Your feelings are validated. You don't have that same sense of isolation, and you don't feel like this difficult experience is just happening to you; there are other people who are going through the same thing. You don't have to explain yourself. You just get to tell your story and watch people nod in agreement. Few things feel better than that. Other caregivers know exactly what to say. They ask the right questions and have answers to your deepest worries. They listen without trying to fix things.

What I've learned from building my community is that I needed to take a leap of faith and trust so I could get the right support. I realized it takes bravery and courage to say the hard things, but it's so important to reveal them. When you do, you take away the power of those thoughts. You lower the shame. You reduce the stigma. You feel less alone.

## QUESTIONS AND ANSWERS WITH PATTI DAVIS

As I mentioned, Patti, whom I look to as a mentor, and I became friends after she so generously sent her book with a card encouraging me to reach out if I needed anything. She's shared such priceless insight with me—in the book and in person—about so many things, especially the importance of support from a community.

**My world opened once I found my people and community. Everything changed for the better almost overnight. Why do you think this is, and why is community so important?**

You need to be around people who are having or had a similar experience. You can forge a connection and obtain much-needed support and you realize that you are part of a very large club. You see that our stories are more alike than different. My experience with my father's Alzheimer's was a very lonely passage because people weren't talking about the disease back then. Once he made the announcement to the world that he had Alzheimer's, sometimes people would recognize me on the street, stop me, and tell me something about their grandmother or parent who had Alzheimer's. But I felt like I was in the French underground; I'd get snippets of information, yet I'd never see that person again and there was no cohesiveness. A decade went on like that, and then after my father passed, I woke up at 3:00 a.m. and thought, *I should start an Alzheimer's caregiver support group.*

When people came into my support groups with their broken places on full display, I knew what that pain felt like. And I knew if they kept coming into that room every week, where it was safe and supportive, where the group members listened to them and didn't judge, they could mend and transform and carve out a new way of living their lives. I started to see people find their footing in a landscape that was changing around them every day. I witnessed people accepting their tears and their pain as tools, not punishment, and finding strength that they didn't know they had.

**I have found that people are so quick to judge. I've been on the receiving side of that. What advice would you give to someone who is experiencing judgment from others?**

Find a community of caregivers. Other people don't mean to be harsh and not understanding; they just don't know any better because they haven't gone through it. Don't talk to those people. Seriously. I don't care if someone is your best friend, if they don't have a loved one who has any form of dementia, don't talk to them about it. I'm not saying don't see them or don't go shopping with them, just don't share this part of your life. When you're a caregiver, you really get down to a very raw place and they're not going to get it. And because you're too vulnerable, if they judge you—even if they just give you a look—you're going to hang on to that for weeks and think that you did something wrong.

## Something to think about . . .

What's one thing you can do to build more community and connection for yourself?

_____

_____

_____

_____

_____

_____

_____

_____

_____

_____

# FOUR

# Make Time for Yourself

It takes great courage to show up for
yourself. You have to do that before you
can show up for anybody else.

**MARIA SHRIVER**

I have seen caregivers run themselves into the ground," Bruce's
doctor said to me early on in the process. "In fact, I've been on
plenty of cases where the caregiver passed away *before* the patient.
Emma, I don't want you to become a statistic."

The statistics he was talking about were sobering: Caregivers die at
a rate that is 63 percent higher than people their age who are not caregivers, and 30 percent of caregivers die before the loved one they are
caring for. This number jumps to 40 percent for caregivers of those
with Alzheimer's and 70 percent for caregivers over the age of seventy.
This is the case even when the care partner is much healthier and has a
lower mortality risk than their loved one.

Hearing this, I was stunned. But that's what happens when extreme
stress builds up over time.

"There may be lots of different diseases with big, complicated
names," says Dr. Habib Sadeghi of Entelechy Medical Center in Los

Angeles. "But when you follow *any* of them back to their roots, there is one common link: chronic stress. That's because long-term stress suppresses immune function, making us more vulnerable to everything from colds to cancer. It doesn't matter if the stress is generated by a job, relationship, health, finances, caregiving, or anything else. Without the ability to neutralize it, over time the emotional fires of life will break us down, create disease, and eventually consume us."

Shortly after Bruce's doctor told me about the rates of caregivers passing away before their loved ones, my stepdaughter Scout approached me. She had noticed my recent chaotic energy and high stress level.

"Emma," she said, "I'm more worried about you than I am my dad." This shook me up even further. *Wow. I'm really losing it*, I thought. *And everyone can see and feel it.*

The truth is, I was just crazed. Steering the course of our future was and remains a balancing act. It still shocks me that I have to make all the major decisions on my own. This is especially difficult because in our family, Bruce was the one who did the heavy lifting, who took things off my plate and made me feel safe, secure, and taken care of. Now I was trying to juggle our kids and Bruce, protect him from the stigma that surrounds cognitive changes, guard our privacy the best I could, and act as if nothing was happening, all at the same time. Honestly, I know that the level of grief, sadness, and stress I experienced has already shaved years off my life. The pace I was going at was not sustainable, and Bruce's doctor, and now my family, knew it.

You see, my go-to is to put everyone's needs above my own (can you relate?), but I've come to realize that doesn't make me a hero. I have always put myself on the bottom of my to-do list, scheduling appointments for my kids and husband but not myself. I'm a perfectionist, striving to do my best and overachieve. While that may sound positive, there is no room for perfectionism in caregiving. In fact, that's a recipe for burnout. The reality is that dementia is a messy disease making it impossible for caregivers to show up perfectly.

Before FTD, Bruce would occasionally talk about someone and say, "He/she just can't get out of his/her own way." I never understood that expression until it hit me in the face: When it came to caring for myself, I was the problem. I planned, organized, and looked after everyone but rarely took time for me. I had stopped exercising, eating right, and getting together with friends. And forget doing anything that would bring me joy, like taking my mom out for lunch and window shopping, or grabbing a coffee and bagel and sitting somewhere peaceful to read the paper. If it came to choosing between doing something for me or taking care of Bruce or my family, I'd choose Bruce and my family every time. *I can't get out of my OWN way*, I realized.

I also wasn't able to make time for our daughters' interests and hobbies. In the early days of Bruce's disease when I was caring for him, I had to bring the girls straight home after school so we could be close to Bruce. To make matters worse, we couldn't host playdates or sleepovers because I was still covering things up and not ready to have these conversations with parents about the challenges we were facing. Would they even feel comfortable leaving their kids at our home? I know I wasn't, because how could I keep my eyes on everything and everyone at one time?

Many of us on the caregiving journey find it hard to take care of ourselves because we're so overwhelmed putting other people's needs above our own. And most of us have no training for this job; instead, you're learning these new skills and putting them to use in real time.

But when you burn the candle at both ends, no one wins. When you spread yourself too thin, it's close to impossible to be your best self for your loved ones. You must refill your cup so that you can be an effective caregiver.

## CARING FOR YOURSELF BENEFITS YOUR LOVED ONE

Refueling and recharging yourself isn't just good for you, it's good for your person. And there's science to prove this. When Dr. Lauren Massimo, associate professor of nursing at the University of Pennsylvania and a researcher in its Frontotemporal Degeneration Center, and her team noticed that FTD caregivers in their clinic were sacrificing their own needs to care for their loved ones, they decided to conduct a study. The premise was that if caregivers intentionally engaged in more restorative activities, they would be in a better place emotionally and physically to look after their loved ones.

Over the course of six months, half of the study participants received ten health coaching sessions that addressed how to cope with stress, sleep, and other issues that would improve their well-being, while the control group received standard care: links to informational websites and occasional outreach from nurses or social workers, but no structured program.

The results were clear. When care partners improved how they looked after themselves, it reduced their levels of stress and depression. But perhaps more surprisingly, behavioral symptoms in the care recipient with FTD improved, too.

"These behavioral changes were significant," says Dr. Massimo.

"There is something called 'stress crossover,' which means that stress doesn't just affect the individual who is experiencing it; it can cross over into your relationship, affecting the other person in a partnership."

This is true for most close relationships. It's certainly true for me when it comes to parenting. I know that my girls feel my negative emotions even if I don't say a word. As Dr. Sadeghi explained to me, those around you are connected to and affected by your emotional Wi-Fi—the mood or presence you bring into a space. And stress crossover is especially prevalent when you're caring for someone with dementia. Your body language and tone of voice tell them exactly how you are feeling. In other words, when you reduce your anxiety and stress, you may lower these emotions in your loved one, too. What a beautiful thing. This is also important because, as Dr. Massimo explains, if your person is anxious and upset, it "might increase symptoms like agitation, disinhibition, or problems communicating effectively."

"The main takeaway is that caring for yourself is important *and* it has downstream effects on your care recipient," she says.

## YOU ARE MORE THAN A CAREGIVER

Not only does taking care of yourself allow you to be a better care partner, but it also helps you to be the best parent, friend, daughter, coworker, fill-in-the-blank that you can be.

"Caregiving is a role, just like motherhood is a role and being a student is a role. It's just a part of you, but it's not the only thing that defines you," explains my therapist, Kathleen Murphy, LMFT. Of course, being a care partner to someone with dementia is a big role and a demanding one, and as a result, it's easy to lose yourself. Early on, in my constant fight-or-flight state, I'd completely lost who I was. Like many care partners, I was so consumed by caregiving that I didn't even know what I liked to do anymore, what made me happy, or even what hobbies I enjoyed.

As advocate, educator, certified dementia practitioner, and caregiver Ty Lewis explains, "A lot of times we get caught up in titles like *I'm a caregiver, I'm an educator, I'm an author, I'm an advocate,* and that becomes your life, and when those things are over, who are you? It's important to not rest in titles but rest in self." Over time, I've come to understand that my responsibilities do not define me.

The good news is that when you realize that caregiving is just a role, you can go deeper to figure out what makes you *you*. This is important to do now so that you feel more fulfilled throughout the journey, can recharge yourself along the way, and are not left feeling even more loss and emptiness once your person has passed.

"Being a care partner isn't a sprint. It's a marathon, and you can't do it without self-care, something that is selfless, not selfish," says Dr. Massimo. "It's about being the healthiest version of yourself so that you can provide the best care possible to your loved one." This is why taking care of ourselves is so important.

In my opinion, the term "self-care" has become overused, and I find it triggering because it's often presented as a one-size-fits-all solution, or packaged as a quick fix that rarely addresses the deeper, more complex, and unique needs we all have. The commercialization of self-care has turned what should be meaningful and personal into something superficial and has created pressure to check off self-care boxes, like going to a spa or doing a face mask, rather than truly tuning in to what we need. Of course, if going to a spa or doing that face mask helps you feel better, that's great. But other things, like a deep conversation with a long-time friend, a creative outlet, or a good night's sleep, may work even better. In fact, that's why my business partner and I named our company Make Time Wellness. First and foremost, it's about getting the world to take women's brain health seriously. Women face a significantly higher risk of cognitive changes than men, yet this issue is often overlooked. But it's also a movement we want women to join so they can identify what truly matters to them and what they want to make time for. (Here's a fun fact: I banned the term "self-care" from our branding at Make Time because that's how strongly I dislike it.)

That said, no matter what you call it, we all need to embrace the importance of recharging and nourishing ourselves on the caregiving journey and in life.

---

"Making time for yourself
can help prevent cognitive decline
and morbidity in caregivers."

**RICHARD S. ISAACSON,**
*MD, founder and director of the Alzheimer's Prevention
Clinic at Weill Cornell Medicine/New York-Presbyterian, the first
of its kind in the United States, and director of research at the Institute
for Neurodegenerative Diseases in Boca Raton, Florida*

---

Reflecting on what Bruce's doctor and Scout said, I vowed that I would do everything in my power not to become a statistic. If I didn't take care of myself, my daughters would end up losing *both* of their parents. No, no, no, I was not going to let that happen. I'm sharing this as your wake-up call. Yes, your loved one has dementia, but it's not your fault, and therefore you cannot allow this disease to take you down with it.

"Just because one person gets the diagnosis doesn't mean both people have to die," says my friend Franne Golde, a former care partner whom you met in Chapter 3.

## MAKING THE TIME

As care partners, we need to do what we can to keep ourselves whole both mentally and physically. I don't have this down to a science at all, but I try. It's a work in progress. Just recently, Evelyn said, "Mom, you need to get out and touch the grass." I knew what she meant. Sometimes I'm wound so tight that she sees and feels it. And this isn't helpful for anyone.

It's taken a while, but now I make a conscious effort to carve out time to take care of myself. For example, when I'm scheduling doctors' appointments for the kids or Bruce, I check my medical notebook to see if I need to make any of my own, because according to Dr. Sadeghi, "one study that found the highest death rates among caregivers revealed 45 percent skipped their own medical appointments because their caregiving did not allow the time." I also make sure I get out of the house and get fresh air, even if it's just for a few minutes, and at least strive to eat healthier and exercise.

Of course, you are devoted to your loved one and want to do right by them. But making time for yourself is an essential part of that devotion. Bruce opened my eyes to what it means to "live it up," as he would say, and encouraged me to do so to the absolute fullest. I know he would want me to get back to living and focusing on my well-being, not sacrifice my health and our daughters' happiness by running myself into the ground. And I think your loved one would want you to consider this as well. So let's talk about what we should be making time for.

## Make Time to Do Things Just for You

If you have the right care in place for your person, I encourage you to start getting out of the house and doing things just for you. This does *not* include picking up prescriptions or grocery shopping. Yes, there was a time when I loved having any errand that got me outside our home, but this is not what experts mean when they talk about how crucial it is to take time for yourself. It also doesn't have to be a fancy spa treatment or weekend away. It's just being intentional about doing things you enjoy as much as possible. Maybe that's running to Starbucks for your favorite drink, soaking in the tub, or going on a hike. Even a walk around the block can shift your mood and mindset. Ask yourself, *What were the simple pleasures I enjoyed prior to becoming a caregiver?* And then make time each day, even if it's just ten minutes, to enjoy them.

## Make Time to Ask for Help

If you don't have help in place that allows you to take time to care for yourself, ask for it, even if it's having someone watch your loved one for an hour or two. You don't need to explain why you need the time or how you plan to spend it. You are entitled to privacy, to step away, and to care for yourself without justification.

The message throughout this book is you can't do this journey alone; that is also the case with making time for yourself. As caregivers, many of us want to handle it all and not feel like a burden to anyone. But the truth is, those in your inner circle *want* to help. Think about how *you* feel when someone you know is going through a rough time. Being a care partner takes a village, so it's important to get used to leaning on others and shift your mindset.

I know it's not easy—I resisted asking for help for a long time. And yes, there have been times when I asked for help and didn't receive it. It doesn't feel good, but don't let that discourage you. If it happens, move on to the next person. Most people truly do want to help. They might just not know how or what to do to be there for you, or they're afraid to ask if they can get involved. But once I let others step in to support me, I felt better and realized that allowing them to contribute gave *them* a sense of purpose, too, and made them feel valued.

Asking for help will also allow *you* to feel some love and attention, which is something we desperately need as care partners. Some experts believe that asking for help strengthens your bond with the other person because you're allowing them to show up for you. As author and inspirational speaker Simon Sinek says, "We don't build trust by offering help, we build trust by asking for it."

To begin asking for help, Katie Brandt, director of caregiver support services at Massachusetts General Hospital's Frontotemporal Disorders Unit, has some recommendations: "Start making a list of all the things that you have to do in your life—cook dinner, mow the lawn, pick up the kids after school, return library books—so that when somebody says, 'If you need anything, let me know,' you can just pull your list out and say, 'Do you want to drop a lasagna off the first Sunday of every month?'"

There are also apps designed to help care partners coordinate assistance from friends and family members. Some even make it easier to ask for help by sending requests directly from the app. When searching for one that fits your needs, look for care coordination apps that allow you to schedule support, share updates, and streamline communication with friends, family, and any others helping you. Keywords like "caregiver task management," "family caregiving support," or "community caregiving organizer" can help you find the right tool. If you don't have time to make a list or use an app, here are a few other suggestions of things friends can do for you:

- Pick up a prescription for you or go on a pharmacy run.

- Go to the grocery store.

- Sit with your loved one for a few hours to give you a break.

- Drive you and your loved one to a doctor's appointment or elsewhere.

- Pick up or drop off your children at school, playdates, or activities.

- Do research for you. This can be related to your loved one, like helping you search for a new doctor or learn about a new medication, or unrelated, like helping you find a good exercise app or a math tutor for your child.

- Make appointments. Again, this could be related to your loved one or unrelated, like scheduling *your* dental, colonoscopy, or mammogram appointments.

And you can also look for help from outside services. Visiting-nurse agencies and respite care services can take over for you for several hours at a time. Faith-based communities may offer some similar services. Community transport services can help get you and your loved one to a doctor's appointment. And don't forget that many grocery stores and pharmacies offer home delivery.

## *Make Time for Your Hobbies*

It's not only okay if you put your needs above everyone else's from time to time, it's necessary. When I think about this, I go back to the metaphor of filling your own cup. When we give so much of ourselves to our loved ones as care partners, parents, friends, etc., we're emptying our cup. Eventually, it will be drained and completely dry. But you can't pour from a vessel that's empty, so it's important to figure out what truly replenishes you. For me, this meant adding layers back to my life that had been slowly taken away by the shift to becoming a caregiver.

The truth is, I didn't even notice these layers were being stripped from my life until one day I looked up and didn't know what made me *me* anymore. I know I'm not alone in this.

"Caregiving situations tend to gradually intensify over time, which is why most caregivers don't realize they're becoming consumed by the increasing demands of the process," says Dr. Sadeghi. "Their normal way of living slowly fades away until they're completely unaware that their new 'normal' is entirely different from the way they used to live. Most of that has to do with the fact that many caregivers don't even have time to think about these differences as they progressively take on more responsibility. Staying aware of your emotions and behaviors while caregiving is essential to know if you're starting to lose yourself in the process."

To remedy this, I began exploring simple things I could do that allowed me to nourish my soul but kept me close to home. This was important because I wasn't comfortable being away from Bruce yet. One of these activities was gardening. First, I claimed part of our garden that I wanted to make my own and learned how to tidy it up. This involved pruning leaves, cutting back branches, and transplanting some of the daisies that were strangling the poppies. Then I bought some new plants and flowers to add to my little plot of land. Soon enough, the garden center became my new happy place and, even though I can't say I have the greenest thumb, tending to these plants and flowers has become my meditation. Going out to the garden in the evenings to water the plants is therapeutic, and watching them grow is so rewarding. But perhaps most beneficial, looking after them is *in my control*, which is a very important feeling for care partners, as we can't control many aspects of our lives.

After taking on gardening and realizing how good it made me feel to learn something new, I looked around our house for things to spruce up. From watching YouTube videos, I learned how to clean and restain our wooden outdoor benches and fence, which got me outside of the house where I could get some fresh air and feel the sun on my face. I was also moving my body and felt a sense of accomplishment because I'd acquired new skills. Listening to music, a podcast, or just the birds chirping while doing these tasks helped me mentally check out just a little. Even though I was still close to home and to Bruce, I was able to find a safe escape. My nervous system settled a bit, and the volume of the stress siren blaring in my head lowered.

"Engaging in hobbies can temporarily pull you out of the chaos of caregiving and rejuvenate you by bringing you joy," says Dr. Massimo. "And having joy and happiness in your life has physiologic effects like reducing the stress hormone cortisol and inflammation. This is important because elevated cortisol and chronic inflammation in the body can lead to heart disease and mortality."

One way to figure out what interests you is to ask yourself, *What were my hobbies before becoming a care partner?* Think about things you loved to do as a child or the extracurriculars you did in high school or college. Was it art, drama, or running track? Then try to include a tiny bit of that in your life. For example, order an adult coloring book, sign up for an online art class, read a new play, or take a ten-minute jog around the neighborhood. Whatever you choose to do should not be overwhelming; it should be fulfilling and give you a mental break from the tunnel vision of caregiving. Start small and set attainable goals. For example, it may not be realistic to exercise for thirty minutes every day, so aim for taking the stairs instead of the elevator, or park in a spot farther away from the store to get in more steps. You might not be able to start a garden right now, but you can spend ten minutes doing some research on the materials you'd need to begin.

One hobby that's relatively easy to get into, is low-cost, and can give you a much-needed escape without requiring you to be away from your loved one is reading.

"When you sit down and read, you can escape to a different world, which can help decrease negative emotions like anxiety and stress and help you feel less alone because you're focused on the stories and lives of others," says Nadine Gaab, associate professor of education at Harvard's Graduate School of Education.

Recently, I got back into reading, as it's something I used to really enjoy but put on the back burner early on in this journey with Bruce. I was so stressed that it was too difficult for me to settle myself enough to focus on anything, let alone pick up a novel and follow a storyline. And forget about retaining anything! So I asked friends to recommend their favorite books and replaced some of my nighttime TV watching with reading. This way, I could get lost in the pages of a great story in the comfort of my own home. Soon reading became a favorite way to check out.

I also love reading books with my girls. We no longer sit and share bedtime stories like we did when they were little, but when they were assigned *The Wild Robot* by Peter Brown for school, we each read it out loud or silently and then talked about it. Escaping the heaviness of our reality into a world that was light and fun was such a relief. (A bonus was when the movie came out and we went to see it together. Any chance to bond with my girls is a good one!)

Also, while I love that you've made time to pick up this book, consider picking up some fiction, too. Don't limit yourself to only reading about dementia. The other night, Mabel was looking at the books on my nightstand and said, "Do you only read books on dementia? Mom, you need to change it up!" Leave it to your child to tell it like it is. Finding balance, even in what we read, is important.

You know what else we need to make time for? Nothing. Our days are so busy and scheduled, but I miss the simplicity of having no plans, a day with an open calendar, so I can just see where it takes me. Those unscripted moments often bring the most joy. Bruce called that "noodling around," and yet it's something I haven't done in a long time. I've got to work on that.

## MAKE TIME TO ENJOY LIFE'S SIMPLE PLEASURES

Feeling overwhelmed and unsure of what to do for yourself? Perhaps the following suggestions will get you started or inspire you.

- Make time to visit the farmer's market.

- Make time to stretch.

- Make time to read.

- Make time to sew, knit, or crochet.

- Make time to learn something new.

- Make time to call your best friend/sister/mom/ fill-in-the-blank.

- Make time to smile.

- Make time to give back.

### Make Time to Move Your Body

Movement is important to help boost your mood and reduce your stress level. It's also crucial for your physical health, something studies show care partners often let fall by the wayside. Yet in the beginning it was something I was not doing enough, partly because I wasn't ready to leave Bruce to take a hike, try an exercise class, or even walk around the block. So I found Melissa Wood-Tepperberg, a fitness expert who has a seemingly endless library of workouts on her app. I could do Pilates and yoga from the comfort of my own home. The workouts are also labeled very specifically by their length, for example, twelve-minute arms and abs, and eleven-minute Power Pilates, so I was able to exercise for as long as I could in that moment. At times I didn't finish the whole twelve minutes, but something was better than nothing. These were the baby steps I took before I was ready to branch out and do an activity away from home.

If you're finding it hard to carve out the time to exercise, don't have the ability to leave your loved one, or don't know where to begin, start small. Do jumping jacks in your living room or put on your favorite music and dance for ten minutes. Or find a short workout video online. There are so many at-home options. Just do what you can, when you can; it's better than nothing, and every small step adds up health-wise and makes you feel stronger and more energized.

Slowly, as I put the right care in place, I worked up to doing things that got me out of the house, like going on a thirty-minute hike. I also started taking tennis lessons and committed to playing one day a week, either in a clinic, which brought me around other people learning to play, or in lessons from a pro. I absolutely loved it. I played tennis earlier in my life but had never learned correct form, like how to hold a racket or properly hit and serve the ball. To unlearn all the bad habits I'd picked up, I needed to be present in those lessons and disconnect from worrying about Bruce and all the responsibilities that waited for me at home. A break I sorely needed to be the best caregiver I could be.

I was also aware that learning a new skill is important for my brain health, so I saw it as a gift to myself. I was thrilled when I read about the Copenhagen City Heart Study, which followed more than 8,500 people over twenty-five years looking at various physical activities and their impact on life expectancy. Results revealed that regularly playing tennis added almost ten years to study participants' lives, which was the most of any of the sports studied.

"People who play racket sports live longer, and because these sports work out your cerebellum, parietal lobes, and frontal lobes, they're great for your whole brain," says Daniel Amen, MD, one of the most influential experts on brain health, founder of the Amen Clinics, and author of several books, including *Change Your Brain Every Day: Simple Daily Practices to Strengthen Your Mind, Memory, Moods, Focus, Energy, Habits, and Relationships.*

Whatever you do to move your body, make it fun, whether that's picking up a sport you used to play (like tennis for me), trying out a new workout class, or walking through your neighborhood. Then schedule it into your routine. Making time to move my body is a nonnegotiable for me now, so I try to write it into my calendar in advance because otherwise I won't do it. We schedule everything else in our lives; why not do the same for improving our well-being?

## Make Time for Music

I love having music playing softly in the background in our home. It always lifts my spirits, and when the house isn't so silent, it allows me to focus on the music rather than getting lost in my dreary thoughts. Plus, there's some science behind the benefits of music.

Borna Bonakdarpour, MD, is an associate professor of neurology at Northwestern University's Feinberg School of Medicine and a cognitive/behavioral neurologist and investigator at Northwestern's Mesulam

Center for Cognitive Neurology and Alzheimer's Disease. He and his team are in their second year of a three-year clinical trial looking at the effects of calming music on patients with dementia and their care partners.

"So far, our results show that such music can decrease the burden of care in caregivers of individuals with dementia," he says. "For this purpose, calming music is recommended." Since "calming" is subjective, choose any music that brings you joy.

Music can also benefit your loved one.

"To reduce agitation/anxiety in the person with dementia, the background music should be slow, soft, and as simple as possible not to overwhelm them. If the goal is to encourage and energize the person with dementia, the music needs to have a faster rhythm and be exciting to them," says Dr. Bonakdarpour.

### Make Time to Be Social

Although the thought of socializing may be unappealing, as we've learned so far, interacting with other people can help nourish and refresh you.

"Social connectedness is a fundamental part of being human," explains Dr. Massimo. "It activates your brain and releases feel-good neurotransmitters like oxytocin and dopamine that are important for our mood and physical health."

Of course, as I know too well, it can be difficult and complicated to take a person with FTD or any form of dementia out of his or her environment, so there may not be a lot of chances for caregivers to socialize outside the home, which can be incredibly isolating. For a long, long time, I didn't socialize at all or only said yes to FTD events, not plans with friends. I'm still not great about this, but I've gotten better.

"If you spend all your time with your loved one, it means your life is totally isolated from social connection and support—two things you need to stay healthy because caregiving is immensely stressful and thus dangerous to your health," explains Dr. Pauline Boss, professor emeritus at the University of Minnesota, who was a caregiver to her husband before he passed away.

I know it's hard, but if you can, arrange help so you have a small window of time to connect with other people, perhaps for lunch or a walk. Or ask a friend to come over for coffee in the morning. Set up Zoom or FaceTime get-togethers. You can also try to make plans with another care partner who gets it.

This is also where a support group can come in. My friend Franne told me about a young-onset group she was a part of when she was caring for her husband, Paul. Every month, the caregivers and their loved ones would get together. This way the care partners could connect while staying close to their person. No one was judging anyone because the whole group just understood. Perhaps you can find a group like this through your neurologist's office or a local support group, or you can create your own.

"At our center, we bring people together and help them partner together. For example, if two men both have wives that are living with dementia, one husband may stay with both wives so the other husband can take a break," explains Teepa Snow, the dementia care specialist we met in Chapter 2.

You'll find more advice on getting help in Chapter 8 so that you can make time to be social.

## *Make Time to Be Guilt-Free*

Look, I know your day is stressful. I know your day is hard, and I know it's easier to tell someone to make time for themselves than it is to *do* it. But I think it's important to acknowledge a major reason many of us find it so hard to take care of ourselves, and that is guilt. This is especially true in a society that doesn't allow caregivers the space we need to replenish our souls. "What about your loved one?" people will say. "They have it worse than you do." (Trust me, I've heard it all in the comment sections.) Of course, that may appear to be true, but when I look at Bruce and where he's presently at in his disease, he seems pretty solid right now. He is in the here and now. So yes, FTD is a terrible disease, and I absolutely hate this for him in every way. But I'll tell you, it's harder on our family than it seems to be on him, and I hear that repeatedly from every expert and specialist I talk to.

We need to change the narrative so we can give caregivers permission to think about themselves. Day-to-day, I'm sure all the attention is understandably directed at your loved one. But from time to time, we need to bring it back to you so you can care for yourself and make this long journey ahead of you sustainable. As I've said before, doing so is not selfish; it is self-preserving.

"It's what allows you to continue caregiving," explains Dr. Boss.

Initially, I felt very guilty about doing anything fun, like taking the kids away for a weekend, without Bruce. I was sad he was not able to join us, especially when we were partaking in something he and I had talked about doing with the girls when they were little. But a few things helped alleviate that guilt.

First, Dr. Boss taught me about "both/and" thinking. This is where two things can be true at once. For example, you can have a social life *and* you can care for your person who is ill. You can be a care partner who is grieving the situation with your loved one *and* be someone who enjoys time with close friends. (You'll read more about this in Chapter 6.)

Second, when I finally did take the girls away, I saw how replenishing, healthy, and important it was for the three of us to get a break from the day-to-day world of FTD and caregiving. They needed to see me making time for myself as well as focusing on them. Otherwise what kind of example was I setting? It's exactly what Bruce would want me to do with our kids. In fact, I know how upset he'd be if he thought we were not living our lives just because I felt guilty. Also, when we come back from any sort of "make-time break," it's better for Bruce, too. As I learned from Dr. Massimo's study, my calmer state of mind makes Bruce, and our children, calmer, too. And remember what Dr. Sadeghi said: Your loved ones are connected to your emotional Wi-Fi.

Something else that's helped me manage my feelings of guilt is realizing that I'm doing the best I can to take care of Bruce. I felt a lot of guilt when I finally had to hire a formal caregiver to help me. I felt like no one could care for him like I could (more on that in Chapter 8), and that I was failing my husband by handing some of his care over to someone else. But my friend Patti Davis gave me some eye-opening insight on this topic, and I want to share it with you: "Yes, your loved one is ill and it's a serious illness, but you didn't give him or her dementia so how does self-punishment make any sense? So you shouldn't have any fun or pleasure because they can't?" She reminded me that going out and enjoying time with my girls, with my friends, or by myself doesn't mean I'm shirking my responsibilities, and it doesn't mean

I don't care about or love Bruce. In fact, it's necessary in order to continue to care for him at the high level I'm striving for, and sacrificing joy and fun in my life doesn't make me a better care partner.

"People caring for loved ones with dementia tend to think that the patient is the important one, and they themselves are not as important. But if you don't put yourself first, then the whole thing falls apart. This make no sense and is a toxic attitude to have about yourself. *Your* health deserves attention, too, and you're going to be a healthier caregiver if you have time for yourself, and care for yourself. Otherwise, you're going to end up in the hospital," Patti says. Remember, you are the MVP in this journey—without you, this ecosystem of care you have set up will fall apart.

When it's framed this way, doesn't it make perfect sense? I agree with Patti; after all, if you're in the hospital, how will you tend to your loved one? I now try to keep her words in the forefront of my mind when the inevitable feeling of guilt starts to rear its ugly head. Whenever that happens to you, consider what my therapist, Kathleen, suggests asking yourself: Would my loved one really want me to live a life without joy? Does that really honor the person?

### Make Time for Life to Happen

As John Lennon sang in "Beautiful Boy," "Life is what happens when you're making other plans." Well, life is also what happens while you're caring for your person who has dementia. Other areas of your world don't stop just because you are caregiving or dealing with something difficult. So I believe that we need to make some space to manage the other challenges that will inevitably arise—a job loss or the death of a loved one—*and* celebrate joyous moments, like the birth of a baby in the family, birthdays, weddings, and graduations.

To be honest, I think this is an area I'm failing miserably at right now. I'm in the midst of raising a preteen and a teen (yikes!). That alone requires my full attention, so I need to continue to work on allowing some space for life to happen. I am not the daughter I want to be to my mom, or the stepmother I would like to be to Bruce's older girls. For so long, I couldn't fathom fitting (or didn't want to fit) another thing onto my plate that didn't pertain to anyone besides Bruce, my girls, or my mom. But my therapist reminds me, "When you support other people, they will support you, and that's how you connect. That's humanity." So I am trying my best to show up more often for things that are meaningful and important. I am learning how to expand more into life, to realize that it's not only okay to celebrate and be there for others besides Bruce, but necessary. For instance, my new tradition for each of my stepdaughters' birthdays is to take them to dinner with just myself and their two young sisters rather than doing a big family get-together. Having the evening to ourselves allows us to connect in a beautiful way. It makes me feel good and gives me a moment to acknowledge how far I've come. Creating the mental space to even think of this new, meaningful tradition reflects the progress I've made.

Think about the friends and family in your life. Can you make time to acknowledge their big and small moments? Perhaps find someone to sit with your person so you can take a friend out for her birthday or even just give him or her a call. Connecting in this way not only shows people you care about them, which strengthens your relationships, but also provides the social interaction and a few non-caregiving-centered moments that *you* need.

———

HERE'S THE GOOD news: "Research shows that caregivers who do not experience high stress *don't* die before the loved ones they care for and don't have a mortality rate any higher than the general public," says Dr. Sadeghi. "It's all about balance." And balance looks like making the time to care for yourself on this incredibly stressful journey, in whatever capacity you have at any given moment.

Because from what I know, we get this one life and that's it. That's why I love the expression "Life is not a dress rehearsal." So make time to have some fun. Live it up. This is a choice I have made because I know Bruce would cosign that. If roles were reversed, he'd be doing the same, and I wouldn't want it any other way for him or our children.

## *Something to think about . . .*

What were some activities you loved doing as a child? Were you an artist or on the swim team? Sometimes these things hold clues to what you would enjoy now.

_____

_____

_____

_____

_____

_____

_____

Which friends or family members are you comfortable inviting over for morning coffee or a walk around the block?

_____

_____

_____

_____

_____

_____

_____

Google activities in your town. Is there an art or crafts fair you can go to? What about the farmer's market? These things don't require a lot of time—you can walk through for ten, twenty, or thirty minutes and come home.

_____

_____

_____

_____

_____

_____

_____

Think about the last time something brought you joy. Was it cooking, baking, or painting? You may not be able to take a class or bake something right now, but you could start reading online or watching videos.

_____

_____

_____

_____

_____

_____

_____

_____

_____

_____

_____

_____

_____

_____

_____

_____

_____

_____

_____

# FIVE

# Focus on Your Brain Health

Our brain health is deeply connected
to our lifestyle choices. By nurturing our bodies with
proper nutrition, exercise, and mental engagement, we
can support cognitive vitality throughout our lives.

**DR. LISA MOSCONI,**
*neuroscientist and director of the Women's*
*Brain Initiative at Weill Cornell Medicine*

Caring for someone with dementia is an act of love, but it's also incredibly demanding emotionally, physically, and mentally. You're constantly making decisions, adapting to changes, and carrying an invisible weight that few truly understand. What's often overlooked is the toll this can take on your own brain health.

Research shows that dementia caregivers face a higher risk for cognitive decline, likely due to prolonged stress, disrupted sleep, and the emotional strain of caregiving. I know that's not what I wanted to hear, and you probably don't either, especially if you're part of the 45 percent of care partners who put their own well-being on the back burner. But here's the good news: The pillars of good brain health are easier to implement than you might think, allowing us to better care for our loved ones while also safeguarding our own well-being.

Now, I might not be able to knock it out of the park seven days a week, but a brain-healthy lifestyle is a goal I strive for. My greatest motivator is seeing what dementia looks like firsthand. It's so painful to watch a loved one's brain change and slowly die that it makes you want to protect your own. I don't want this disease, so why not do whatever may be in my control to prevent it? This is my "why." I also do not want our children to go through this experience twice.

To be very clear, FTD is a rare disease, and there was nothing Bruce could have done to prevent it or alter its course. However, there was a period before Bruce was diagnosed when we adopted a brain-healthy lifestyle. During that time, I noticed some improvements, particularly in myself because I was experiencing an alarming amount of brain fog due to stress and hormone shifts. To me, it was empowering to learn that we can positively impact our brains through simple lifestyle changes at any age.

Prioritizing your brain health may seem daunting in the midst of everything else you're navigating at the moment. And like me, you might not be able to give it your all every single day. But taking steps to practice good brain health will not only help you better care for your loved one, it will improve your own life.

---

"If you have kids, you want them
to see you taking care of your brain *and* you
want to take care of their brains so they have these
habits when they're grown up and on their own."

**DR. ANNIE FENN,**
*physician, chef, and author of* The Brain Health Kitchen:
Preventing Alzheimer's Through Food

---

## BRAIN FIRST

I've always been pretty up-to-date on the best wellness practices and ways I need to look after myself. I knew the importance of maintaining my heart, breast, and gut health. But I never knew much about brain health until I met Richard S. Isaacson, a pioneering neurologist whose focus is the treatment and prevention of Alzheimer's disease. Dr. Isaacson founded and directed the Alzheimer's Prevention Clinic at Weill Cornell Medicine/NewYork-Presbyterian, the first of its kind in the United States. Today, he conducts clinical and translational research at the Institute for Neurodegenerative Diseases (IND) in Boca Raton, Florida.

Throughout my journey with Bruce, I'd consulted several neurologists who were brilliant, but Dr. Isaacson was the only one who talked to me about how to support the brain, an organ that is forever changing and aging. Learning this was an aha moment for me. In fact, it's still shocking that my primary care doctor doesn't talk to me about my cognitive/brain health when I go in for my annual exam, particularly since women are at a higher risk of developing dementia than men, and there are preventative measures we can take.

"When someone has a diagnosis of dementia, that means the dementia really started ten, twenty, thirty years before," Dr. Isaacson explains. "While there's no cure for this disease, there is value in looking after our brains—especially because recent studies show that 45 to 50 percent of dementia cases may be preventable by adopting specific health habits. I don't want to overpromise, but I believe that we can make an impact on our brains today, and the earlier you start the better."

Kellyann Niotis, MD, director of Parkinson's and Lewy body dementia prevention research at the IND and its Parkinson's & Alzheimer's Research and Education Foundation, adds, "Our genes are not our destiny and the earlier these dementia risk factors are addressed, the better. That said, there's plenty of evidence here to show that it's never too late to reduce dementia risk."

Today, my approach to my overall health is to think about my brain first, then my whole-body benefits. (In fact, learning about brain health had such a profound effect on me that it inspired me to cofound my wellness brand called Make Time.) I don't do it all perfectly, but for the most part, every day I ask myself, *What did I do for my brain today?* It's not always easy, especially when you're busy caregiving, but supporting our brains is not out of reach. In fact, it's crucial. Why?

"The brain is the most complex structure known to humankind," says Dr. Wendy A. Suzuki, professor of neural science and psychology at NYU and an internationally renowned expert in mental health and brain plasticity. "Our brains define who we are as people—our talents, sense of humor, how we see, feel, and think about the world. And the longer that you keep that brain healthy and happy, the longer you're *you*."

So, let's get into the specific pillars of great brain health.

---

"At any moment and at any time, we can make an impact on brain health. For example, a pregnant mother's diet rich in B vitamins is tied to better cognitive outcomes for her child decades later. Then there are early life, midlife, and late life risk factors for cognitive decline and dementia."

DR. RICHARD S. ISAACSON

---

## NUTRITION

When I say I don't practice brain health perfectly, I'm mostly talking about nutrition. This is often my downfall.

I've always appreciated good food and never really had to watch what I ate. We frequently hear stories about models starving themselves and sometimes becoming anorexic to fit into that size 0, but thanks to genetics, I was naturally slender, so my diet wasn't an issue during my modeling career. However, when I got into my late thirties, and especially after the birth of our second child, Evelyn, I had a hard time losing those extra pounds. Then, over time, with the added stress of the underlying issue that I thought was brewing in my marriage, food became a friend.

What I have come to realize about myself during the process of becoming a caregiver is that I'm an emotional stress eater. There was a point on this journey where I was so stressed that I lost weight, but for the most part, food is my comfort. Growing up, my mom was a great cook and she always made sure to put healthy options on my plate. But I am a child of the '80s and '90s, and left to my own devices, I would happily gravitate toward some childhood favorites: Kraft Mac & Cheese, Carl's Jr., and Snickers bars. (Although back in the day, Snickers were considered good-for-you fuel due to very strategic marketing!)

Over the years, all the traveling I did as a model thankfully helped me expand my palate, but there's nothing like grief and sadness to make you reach for the things that give you instant pleasure. So in those tough moments I can easily revert to my childhood diet for some comfort. This is what I did in those early years of caregiving for Bruce. I also wasn't moving my body like I should have because I was so busy with our two young daughters, worrying about Bruce, and working. My whole life was upside down, and the motivation to do anything for my health was just not there.

However, once I understood that what was happening to Bruce was serious, I realized it was important for me to get my act together when it came to nutrition. I wanted to be healthy for myself and our children, and to be able to take care of Bruce and make clear-headed decisions on his behalf. And of course, the statistic I mentioned in the previous chapter about care partners dying before the person they care for, which various studies reveal can be as high as 63 percent, motivated me to change my eating habits as well. Once I altered what I was putting into my body, I started to see an improvement in my energy level and a reduction in some brain fog that I was experiencing.

I also learned more about the gut-brain connection, or the link between what you eat and how well your brain works. In fact, experts call the gut our second brain. While too much processed food and sugar can make you feel sluggish and foggy, eating fiber, good fats, and probiotic-rich foods—like sauerkraut, pickles, and other fermented things—can help reduce stress and inflammation by supporting your gut health. These foods also help your brain function and overall well-being.

"Hundreds of studies show that the Mediterranean diet is healthy for both the heart and brain," explains Dr. Annie Fenn, author of *The Brain Health Kitchen: Preventing Alzheimer's Through Food*, a science-based cookbook and care manual for the brain. This lifestyle diet, which is also known to reduce inflammation, is centered around nutrient-dense fruits, vegetables, whole grains, nuts, fish, and olive oil, while limiting processed foods, red meat, and added sugars. Although my goal is to follow the Mediterranean diet 100 percent of the time, it's really more like 70 percent because a girl's gotta live and find joy, too!

The Mediterranean-DASH Intervention for Neurodegenerative Delay (MIND) diet study published in 2015 was the first to show that following a brain-protective dietary pattern could significantly reduce Alzheimer's risk. For four and a half years, researchers tracked almost eight hundred people who did not have dementia and instructed them to follow the MIND diet, a variation on the Mediterranean pattern of eating tailored to be more brain-focused. It has nine food groups: berries, leafy greens, vegetables, nuts, beans and legumes, whole grains, fish and seafood, poultry, and extra virgin olive oil. Study participants who followed the MIND diet closely, scoring in the upper third for adherence by regularly eating brain-healthy foods, had a 53 percent reduction in being diagnosed with Alzheimer's, which is equivalent to being 7.5 years younger. And these people were in their fifties, sixties, and seventies, age groups where one is at higher risk for this disease. Importantly, the *only* thing they changed over the course of those four and a half years was their diet.

The MIND diet also benefited those who didn't adhere to it as strictly. Those who followed it about half the time still had a 35 percent reduction in their Alzheimer's risk.

"Since then, the study has been replicated in other countries and shown the same results," explains Dr. Fenn. "In terms of brain health, people who follow the MIND and Mediterranean diets have less plaque and tau tangles in their brain." (Tau tangles are an abnormal accumulation of protein in brain neurons found in Alzheimer's disease.) The MIND diet has also been shown to reduce the risk of Parkinson's and breast cancer, among other diseases. Another study showed that if you eat leafy greens about once a day, over the course of time, your brain looks eleven years younger in an MRI compared to someone who rarely eats a salad.

When I spoke to Dr. Fenn about the ideal brain-healthy diet, she gave me the following tips for changing how you eat:

### First, change your mindset.

Ask yourself, *Why do you want to take care of your brain? What is it that you're trying to achieve?* For example, do you want to be a healthy grandmother who can run around with your grandchildren well into your seventies and eighties? Do you want to be able to travel? Do you want to pursue the work you're doing for many more years? Do you want to prevent the dementia that is stealing so much from a loved one? That's your "why." By grounding your intention to eat this way in a bigger sense of purpose, you're less likely to go back to your old habits.

### Eat the rainbow.

We've heard this before, but a colorful diet is important because the various colors in fruits and vegetables represent different plant pigments called flavonoids, which are brain-healthy nutrients. To add more color to your plate, Dr. Fenn suggests trying new fruits and veggies every week, maybe starting with variations of those you already eat. For example, if you always buy white cauliflower, try the purple one. If you typically get red tomatoes, try yellow ones.

### When it comes to oils, stick with extra virgin olive oil.

"Most of the oils that you see at the supermarket are highly, highly processed, which means they've been changed in a way that can be harmful to our blood vessels," says Dr. Fenn. Extra virgin olive oil, however, has the perfect fat content for a brain-healthy diet: mostly monounsaturated fats, with some polyunsaturated fats and a small proportion of saturated fat.

"Olive oil is also high in polyphenols, which reduce oxidative stress and quell inflammation in the brain. No other oils stack up in terms of how much scientific data is behind it," says Dr. Fenn.

### Don't cook on high heat.

"Cooking in a really hot pan creates inflammatory advanced glycation end products that are bad for brain cells and associated with Alzheimer's," says Dr. Fenn. The best cooking techniques are low and slow. Steam and braise rather than sear, since this is a technique that requires cooking food at high temps.

### Limit or avoid foods that accelerate cognitive decline.

Stay away from foods high in saturated fat, trans fats, and excess sugar.

"Avoid sugary foods that don't have any fiber—like soda and candy. This is the most harmful way to consume sugar because it goes right to your bloodstream and can trigger a spike in insulin and lead to insulin resistance, which we know is one of the precursors to getting Alzheimer's," explains Dr. Fenn. Monk fruit, stevia, dates, maple syrup, and honey are good replacements, and even brown sugar is fine if it's in something that contains fiber.

"Avoid all processed meats (which have been strongly linked to dementia), and limit unprocessed meat to no more than three small (under three ounce) portions a week," says Dr. Fenn. Limit cheese to no more than an ounce a week, butter to less than a tablespoon a day, fried food only once a week, and under five servings of sweets a week.

### *Drink low or moderate amounts of alcohol.*

I've always appreciated a glass of red wine with dinner and love the whole ritual of pairing wine with food because I am a foodie at heart. I was never a hard alcohol person, but then I noticed I was branching out and having margaritas in the summer and cold sake with sushi. Dinner and a drink became a habit. To be perfectly honest, I liked how it slowed my habit of overthinking and the swirling thoughts in my mind, and helped take the edge off my grief and sadness. However, when I acknowledged that, I realized I was on a slippery slope. I don't have the gene linked to alcoholism, and I can have one drink and stop. But as Dr. Fenn reminded me, "We have so much data saying that alcohol is not as good for our brains as we once thought, and it actually increases the risk of dementia."

Even a single drink, night after night, is probably not healthy, and when it comes to the brain specifically, a glass of red wine just isn't that beneficial. I also realized that having a drink disrupted my sleep so I didn't feel my best in the morning. It just wasn't worth it to me, so I decided to cut back. I don't want to be too rigid around it and will have a drink for celebratory occasions, but I've found that I'm perfectly happy making mocktails for myself and the girls that we can all enjoy. There are also so many delicious nonalcoholic choices on restaurant menus these days. (Although you do have to watch for those filled with sugar.)

Since cutting my alcohol intake by 90 percent, I sleep better and feel more alert during the day. And it sounds like my brain benefits, too.

### Sip your coffee and tea.

"Huge population studies from coffee-drinking cultures—like Europe— show that drinking coffee reduces dementia risk," says Dr. Fenn. Coffee and green, white, black, and oolong teas are high in polyphenols, which are neuroprotective.

"Just make sure you don't make this brain-healthy drink unhealthy by the things that you add to it—like a lot of sugar and creamers," she says. A splash of nut milk is your best bet.

### Make small swaps.

If this is starting to feel overwhelming, know that you don't need to totally revamp your diet.

"When you try to improve your dietary patterns, look at what you eat on a daily basis and then upgrade it," Dr. Fenn suggests. For example, if you have toast for breakfast every day, choose whole-grain bread instead of white and swap your usual butter for olive oil or almond butter.

### Remember, eating for brain health is a lifestyle, not a diet.

"This is not something you're going on in January and then going off in February. It's about folding these proven neuroprotective foods into the way you eat and live," says Dr. Fenn. To make eating brain-healthy foods easier, I try to keep our pantry and refrigerator stocked. If I don't, I'll grab something unhealthy when I'm in a rush or hungry.

Dr. Fenn suggests filling the kitchen with minimally processed foods like salsa verde (one with a short, clean ingredients list), cans of black beans and cannellini beans, hummus, frozen vegetables like butternut squash and corn, and frozen fruit like berries, which you can blend for a dessert or smoothie or add to yogurt.

"Sometimes frozen fruits and vegetables are better than fresh because they're frozen at the peak of ripeness," explains Dr. Fenn.

Plan your meals and snacks ahead of time so you're not left scrambling when hunger strikes, whether you're running errands, at a long doctor's appointment, or in between caregiving tasks. Good options include small containers of hummus with carrot sticks, nuts, medjool dates, single-serve almond butter packets, homemade granola or store-bought with few ingredients, hard-boiled eggs, and sachets of green tea. Keeping a few of these on hand in your bag or car can help sustain you throughout the day, making it easier to nourish yourself even in the busiest moments.

Also, since it's hard to stick to a perfect diet, some experts suggest taking supplements to fill the gaps. Dr. Fenn says you can't go wrong with a multivitamin, and Dr. Isaacson recommends omega-3 fatty acids, vitamin B complex, and vitamin D. Check with your doctor before taking these or any supplements.

# Omega-Boost Energy Bites

These are quick to prepare, require no baking, and provide you with sustained energy and focus while promoting brain health. I love them and so do my kids.

INGREDIENTS:

1 cup rolled oats (supports sustained energy and brain function)

¼ cup ground flaxseed (rich in omega-3 fatty acids for brain health)

½ cup nut butter (almond or peanut butter for healthy fats and protein)

(Optional) ¼ cup dark chocolate chips or chopped nuts (for an extra treat and crunch)

INSTRUCTIONS:

In a medium bowl, mix all the ingredients until well combined.

Put a piece of parchment paper on a baking sheet.

Roll into 1-inch balls using your hands.

Place balls on the parchment and refrigerate for 15–20 minutes to firm up.

Store in an airtight container in the fridge for up to a week.

## EXERCISE

We talked in the previous chapter about some of the benefits of movement when it comes to taking care of yourself. But experts also say that regular exercise is the number-one thing you can do for brain health, both in the short and long term.

"Exercise lowers a sticky plaque called amyloid, which is a pathologic protein that builds up in the brains of people with Alzheimer's, Lewy body dementia, and other diseases," says Dr. Isaacson.

"In the short term, exercise releases a bubble bath of neurochemicals in the brain—dopamine, serotonin, and adrenaline—that have an immediate effect," adds Dr. Suzuki. "This means that every time you move your body—even during a ten-minute walk—these neurochemicals help reduce anxiety and depression and increase your energy levels. Moving your body regularly can improve your mood state over time because you're bringing those chemicals into your life consistently. It also releases growth factors, which can help build new brain cells in the hippocampus and new synapses in your prefrontal cortex."

I asked Dr. Isaacson and Dr. Suzuki for their exercise tips. Here's what they had to say:

### *Start small and move when you can.*

When I first got back into the idea of exercise while caregiving for Bruce, there were times when five minutes was all I could manage. But that's okay, because as Dr. Isaacson says, "Five minutes of exercise is better than zero, ten minutes is better than five, and so on."

Over time, I was able to level up and work out longer. One thing that's helped? Apps. As I mentioned in Chapter 4, I love an app called Melissa Wood Health, which has short Pilates and yoga strength workouts I can squeeze in anywhere. They're labeled by their duration so you can find one that fits into an opening in your schedule, no matter how brief. (The app also has meditations that you can use if you can't muster up the energy for a workout and what you really need is to relax your mind. Doing something for your mental health is important, too.)

Although I know it's less convenient when you're a care partner, there is also something to be said about an in-person fitness class environment. One, it gets you out of the house, and two, once you're in that class, you are (hopefully) just focused on whatever exercise you need to do within that forty-five to sixty minutes rather than thinking about your loved one. A third benefit is the social interaction, which is another pillar to maintaining a healthy brain (more on that in a second). On days when I need extra motivation, I remind myself how lucky I am to be able to move my body, and that I want to hold on to that ability as long as possible.

### *At a minimum, increase your physical activity.*

You don't need to take an exercise class to reap the brain-health benefits of movement. Simply moving your body in ways that fit your life right now is a great place to start, whether it's pushing a wheelchair, folding laundry, brushing the dog, or gardening. These activities count, especially when done with intention. But as you're able, consider gradually expanding into more structured forms of exercise, even if it's just dancing in the kitchen or gentle stretching. Every bit of movement matters.

Walking is also helpful. A study of over seventy-eight thousand people published in the *Journal of the American Medical Association Neurology* found that people who walked around ten thousand steps per day, which is about five miles, reduced their risk of developing dementia by 51 percent. Even those who did just 3,800 steps, about two miles, reduced their risk by 25 percent.

Other research shows that walking may enhance the health of your brain neurons. A brisk pace, one where you can talk but not easily, is best, but any walking helps.

"This is especially the case after a meal, where it can aid digestion, move sugars out of the bloodstream, and speed up your metabolism," says Dr. Isaacson. Even a quick five to ten minutes or a stroll around the block is a good idea. Recently, I purchased a weighted vest to increase the intensity of my walks. The benefits of adding this include increasing bone density and improving cardiovascular health, muscular endurance, and posture.

### *If you can, shoot for physical exercise.*

When it comes to physical exercise, the ideal is to try to do a little cardiovascular exercise, strength training, and stretching each week.

There are two types of cardiovascular exercise. High-intensity interval training, done with a doctor's permission, helps condition the body and strengthen the heart. "This can be twenty minutes, thirty minutes, forty minutes," says Dr. Isaacson.

Then there is lower-intensity cardio, which Dr. Isaacson calls Zone Two. This is when your heart rate is around 60 to 70 percent of your maximum. Calculate this by subtracting your age from 220 and multiplying the result by 0.6 to 0.7. In this zone, you can carry a conversation, but it's difficult.

"As your belly size gets larger, the memory center in the brain gets smaller. As long as you can tolerate it—and check with your doctor before doing any exercise—forty to forty-five minutes two to three times a week will help you burn fat, which impacts your risk of dementia," says Dr. Isaacson.

Strength training is also important, and there are so many ways you can do this, from equipment-free exercises like push-ups, sit-ups, and tricep dips to using free weights.

"Building muscle mass can improve metabolic health—things like insulin resistance—and metabolism is linked to memory dysfunction," Dr. Isaacson says.

Stretching improves your mobility and flexibility, which are important for the health of your joints and injury prevention. It also helps bring nutrients to your muscles while removing any toxins.


### Find what works for you.

The key to exercising regularly is finding things you like to do that are sustainable.

"You also don't want to get hurt so if you don't know anything about exercise, learn about it. Work with a personal trainer. Obviously, there's a cost to that, but it's so important to stay active," adds Dr. Isaacson.

Hiking is a favorite workout of mine because it gets me out into nature. There was one trail close to our home that was about twenty-five minutes up on a steady-ish incline and twenty minutes down. (Unfortunately, it was lost in the Palisades Fire in January 2025.) In the early days, the thought of being away from home and Bruce for that long was too stressful for me, so it took a while for me to branch out. But when I finally hit that trail, it was worth it. Getting outside with the sun on my face just feels good to me. I've done some of my best creative thinking and problem-solving on those hikes. And as you know, there's a lot of creative thinking and problem-solving that needs to be done when it comes to caregiving. Having some separation from the home and my loved ones also helps me think clearly, shifts my perspective, and allows me to manage feelings of overwhelm.

As I mentioned in Chapter 4, I also take tennis lessons and play when I can. I love that it's such a technical sport, and experts say that tennis is excellent for your brain health because it works your cerebellum, parietal lobes, and frontal cortex. It's also rewarding to see my game improve. Plus, there's the social aspect, which is beneficial, too. Occasionally, I like to join clinics because you get to play with other people. Sometimes with women in their sixties and seventies running circles around me! Also, you don't have to be part of a country club to play tennis. In my neighborhood there are community courts that have a bulletin board where you can find names of group clinics and local tennis instructors.

It might take a little trial and error to see what type of exercise brings you joy and helps you feel those mood-boosting endorphins, but once you do, you'll actually look forward to it. I know I do.

## Set realistic goals and mix it up.

With everything that's going on in my life, I'm not doing fifty to sixty minutes of exercise every day. Instead, I set realistic goals. For me, this is exercising at least three times a week for thirty minutes—any more than that is a bonus. As I mentioned before, this hasn't always been the case. For years, I did next to nothing, then I'd go through phases where I'd push too hard and get burned out. Not only was this cycle exhausting, but it wasn't really sustainable.

What's also helped me to become more consistent is mixing it up with a variety of physical activities, like hiking, spinning, tennis, walking, and working with a personal trainer who specializes in functional training. This is when you do exercises that strengthen your body for everyday movements, such as carrying and lifting heavy things and climbing stairs.

I know finding this time might be challenging. Here are some ideas for making it work: Is there room in your home to bring in a piece of workout equipment, like a treadmill or a stationary bike? Do you think using one of the workout apps we've talked about might be a good place to start and build upon? (Some TVs allow you to stream or screen mirror these apps.) Or how about just setting a goal for yourself, like doing ten push-ups (starting with one good one a day) or five minutes of going up and down the stairs (starting with just one minute)? How about a walk around the block? For instance, I'm working on being able to do the splits. Right now, it's pretty laughable and extremely painful, but I will get there!

## SLEEP

"Exercise loosens that sticky plaque in the brain and sleep takes this trash out," says Dr. Isaacson. "However, sleep is one of the hardest things for caregivers to manage because you're on 24/7, and the person with dementia doesn't have normal functioning circadian rhythms."

Not only does this mean that they're up in the night, but their disturbed sleep can disturb you and often this happens long before you realize that caregiving is your new role. This was definitely the case for me.

As Bruce's disease progressed, the eight to nine hours of shut-eye I needed to feel good and rested became nonexistent. It reminded me of becoming a mother, when you go from being a sound sleeper to someone who wakes up at the slightest sound. I felt like I had to sleep with one eye open because I was worried about everyone's safety in the middle of the night if Bruce was restless. Relaxing and switching my mind off wasn't easy.

I'm sure you can relate to this feeling that you may be called into action at any second. Unfortunately, this creates a vicious cycle because sleep deprivation is bad for your physical health (like your brain and heart, for example), mood, ability to cope with stress, and productivity, and all of this makes it harder to caregive.

Dr. Isaacson recommends trying to get at least one or two full nights of sleep per week.

"It's not going to solve the problem, but it can vastly reduce the impact on morbidity and chronic health conditions for caregivers," he says.

How do you ensure a few nights of good sleep?


### *Create a dementia-friendly home.*

One way to rest a little easier is to adapt your home for the safety of your loved one. (After all, if your person's brain is degenerating, he or she is not thinking about safety, so that's your job now.) For example, your stove should have childproof knobs, your refrigerator and freezer should be locked so they can't be accidentally left open, and all doors should be secured so your person can't wander out.

### Get a nighttime caregiver.

If possible, try to arrange for a nighttime caregiver. While there are costs involved and it can feel challenging to ask friends or family members to cover the night shift, reaching out for occasional help, even if just one or two nights a week, can make a meaningful difference in your sleep. The investment, whether financial or logistical, may provide much-needed rest and allow you to better care for your loved one during the day.

At some point, I had to hire someone, not only so I could sleep and be fresh for our children in the morning, but for the safety of our household. I held off on doing this for as long as I could. I yearned for our old life and normalcy; this was yet another thing that made everything in my world feel so foreign. I also really valued our privacy, and the thought of having someone in our sacred space at night while we slept didn't sit right with me. But I considered it when Bruce's neurologist told me that not having someone to help at night was posing a potential safety hazard for everyone in the house, and that it was bad for my own health to have such disrupted sleep. I needed to hear that and was so grateful to Bruce's neurologist for that reminder. (More on this in Chapter 8.)

### Create a sleep routine.

When you *do* have time to get some shut-eye, Dr. Isaacson suggests getting off your phone at least thirty minutes before going to bed because the blue light can artificially suppress melatonin, a hormone you need to sleep. He also recommends creating a bedtime routine to send a signal to your body that it's time to sleep. My routine helps relax my nervous system. It includes taking a gummy supplement to ease myself into sleep, using an essential-oil lavender pillow spray, turning on my aromatherapy diffuser, slowing my breathing, and journaling or reading a book. I really set the mood, so I don't just slam myself into bed. Your routine might include a meditation or special blanket you only use while sleeping. If possible, try to go to bed at the same time every night, too.

### Squeeze sleep in whenever you can.

Another suggestion I've heard is what experts recommend for new parents: nap when your person naps. Of course, this isn't always easy since you have so many things you probably want to do in that "free" time, but experiment with how this makes you feel. A little sleep here and there is better than none.

## REDUCE YOUR STRESS

Being a caregiver means walking through something that is incredibly distressing. Every. Single. Day. To me, it felt as if a siren was going off next to my ear 24/7. As I've mentioned in other parts of the book, we need to reduce that stress response and protect ourselves from chronic stress even when we're living this life. The pitfalls can be devastating.

"Chronic stress causes inflammation throughout the body, and inflammation fast-forwards aging—both brain aging and body aging," says Dr. Isaacson.

"Plus, chronic stress can literally shrink the brain, damaging brain cells in the hippocampus and prefrontal cortex, two important areas that are very severely affected in frontotemporal dementia," adds Dr. Suzuki.

As we talked about earlier, this could contribute to why caregivers of people with Alzheimer's or other types of dementia pass away earlier than the person they're caring for and, on average, die at a younger age than non-caregivers. I'm not trying to alarm you, but hearing these hard truths and statistics was the wake-up call I needed to shift gears.

"Stress reduction comes in many forms, so it has to be what you're most interested in and what resonates with you," says Dr. Isaacson.

Here are some stress-reduction strategies to explore:

### Talk to someone.

I'm a fan of talk therapy. The ability to share my thoughts and express *all* my feelings in a safe, confidential space without judgment has greatly reduced my stress level. (Journaling also helps me with this.) My therapist keeps me in check and accountable to make sure I'm looking after myself.

A support group is a great place to express yourself, too. (See Chapter 3 for more on this.) And if you don't have time to do this in person, Dr. Isaacson suggests using technology. "You can also reduce stress by having a meaningful interaction via text message, phone, or video."

### Meditate and breathe.

A consistent meditation practice helps with stress relief because you can shift from reacting to choosing, and living a life rooted in choice rather than reaction changes everything. Now, for me, this is easier said than done. I'm learning how to meditate, but being still and silent can be difficult because that's when dark, scary thoughts start creeping into my head, and my cycle of what-ifs and catastrophizing begins. I feel myself spiraling.

I used to see this as a negative but what I've learned is that it's okay. Some days, meditation brings peace; other days, it doesn't. The practice isn't about erasing your thoughts; it's about learning to notice and separate yourself from them so you don't get caught in their swirl. Let go of the idea that you need to be like a Buddha on a mountaintop with a perfectly clear mind. Meditation is about progress, not perfection.

There are times in my Meditation 101 practice where I pull myself out of that dark place by literally shaking these thoughts off and focusing on breathing slowly and using mantras like "I inhale peace and exhale worry." This stabilizes my racing heart and helps me envision the words I'm reciting in my head. Or, as my mind begins to spin, I tell myself, "Stay here, don't go there." This keeps me in the present moment.

"When your nervous system is activated, it's primed to see danger everywhere," explains my therapist, Kathleen. "So the alarm goes off in your head and then a story starts in your mind through the lens of 'We're all in danger.' Telling yourself, 'Stay here, don't go there' helps you be with what is and prevents you from borrowing tomorrow's troubles today."

There is something to be said for taking it day by day or even hour by hour. It brings you to the present. One form of meditation therapy that can help with this mindset is called mindfulness-based stress reduction (MBSR), an evidence-based program developed by Dr. Jon

Kabat-Zinn. It's a combination of mindfulness meditation, body aware-ness, and gentle movement. The goal is to help reduce stress and pain and manage your emotions. Essentially, you focus on observing your thoughts and emotions without reacting to them. This allows you to cultivate a sense of calm even in the midst of caregiving stress.

"It's a structured way to be more resilient to stress," explains Dr. Isaacson.

If you want to learn more about MBSR, I highly recommend *Full Catastrophe Living: Using the Wisdom of Your Body and Mind to Face Stress, Pain, and Illness* by Jon Kabat-Zinn. It's a great resource for anyone looking to bring more calm, balance, and resilience into their caregiving journey. You can also find videos about MBSR online.

Even if you can't meditate, Dr. Isaacson suggests that you stop and take three slow deep breaths twice a day.

"You can do this anytime—when you're washing your hands, going to the bathroom, right before bed, or on line at the store," he explains. My therapist has me set an alarm on my phone that goes off four times during the day. When it does, I must stop, feel the state of my body, lower my shoulders (which are usually around my ears), and take some in-the-moment cleansing breaths. It's always interesting (and sad) to see how much tension is being held in my body prior to the alarm going off. But if I didn't have that reminder, I'd be in stress mode all day long, and I don't want to live like that. I'm sure you don't either.

Try setting your alarm to remind yourself to breathe. This is a sim-ple way of helping you rebalance and regulate yourself a few times a day.

### Get moving.

Not only is physical movement important for your health, but as we discussed in the last chapter, it's also great for stress reduction. Gardening has become a form of meditation for me, and at times, even home improvement projects and upkeep can work. These things allowed me to stay close to home while being safely removed and outdoors. There is no longer a "man of the house," so I've stepped up and it's empowering. And I like that our two daughters can see all the things women are capable of. We don't fall into a box. Sure, I can call in a handyman and gardeners, but I like learning something new and being hands-on with a project. It gets me out of my head and focused on something besides FTD and caregiving.

So what about you? Are there projects or hobbies you can safely do around your home or that can get you outside and moving?

### Get some respite.

I'd never heard of respite care until Bruce's diagnosis. Respite care is when you're able to get away for a night, weekend, or week. Although this may require a lot of organization, it's important for reducing chronic stress.

"Without it, people break themselves, and getting broken doesn't change dementia, it just breaks another human being," Teepa Snow explains. When Teepa said this to me, it gave me chills and made me emotional. I *still* get emotional thinking about it because taking time away from Bruce has always hit a chord of guilt and shame in me. It's brought up intense feelings of thinking I'm less than, and that I wasn't properly fulfilling my spousal commitment and simply just failing as a care partner. But I also knew I was breaking. And that certainly doesn't help me, Bruce, or our two daughters who rely on me for their care.

"By stepping away and creating a safe space for yourself you're getting true respite," Teepa explains. "During that time, truly give yourself permission to let go of being a carer and simply be a human being for a little while." Reach out to family and friends to see if they can be with your person so you can get a break. You can also look into some of the organizations for your person's disease and see if they offer any respite grants. (Find some suggestions on my website, emmahemingwillis.com.)

### Ask for help.

At this point in this book, you know that you can't caregive alone. This is essential for stress reduction. You need to accept that you're going to need help in one way or another at some point, and that it's okay.

"Asking for help is a dirty word in the caregiving space because people think it means that they're giving up or not a good spouse/partner/daughter," says Dr. Isaacson. "But for your loved one's safety and well-being, not letting everything fall on your own shoulders is critical. If you don't take care of yourself, how can you take care of the person you love? So be realistic and ask for help earlier than later. Nine times out of ten, people wait way too long."

Of course, asking for help is easier said than done, and I know it can be challenging for any of us who lack the support of family and friends or the resources to hire help. If you're facing that scenario, think about the people in your inner circle and ask yourself these questions: Who is your loved one comfortable with? Who recently told you, "If you need anything, let me know"? Take them up on it. Friends may be willing to take on the night shift or financially contribute to hiring someone.

"When you take a respite, you just need to know that the individual is getting some care; it may not be the best care, it may not be *your* care, but it's better than you *not* taking a break," says Teepa. (For more on the topic of bringing in help, see Chapter 8.)

### *Write it out.*

Various studies show that journaling can help reduce stress and anxiety, analyze your emotions, and break the cycle of negative thinking, among other things that improve your well-being. In fact, one of the unexpected benefits of writing this book was learning how healing and therapeutic writing can be. One technique I used was to set my timer for seven minutes and just put my thoughts on paper, either with a writing prompt to guide me or without one.

## STAY SOCIALLY CONNECTED

Another pillar of brain health is making sure to stay cognitively engaged.

"There's so much research behind the power of social connection and its link to longevity. The more social connections you have, the longer your life. Why? Because we are social animals, and we have so many circuits in our brain that have evolved to be in social situations," says Dr. Suzuki.

This has motivated me to work on being more connected to others, both for my sake and Bruce's. In the beginning, I lied to friends about why Bruce and I wouldn't be able to join them because I didn't want them to sense that something was off with him and how uncomfortable I was. Now that I understand the importance of social interaction, and Bruce and I are more settled in his disease, I push myself outside of my comfort zone and seek out time to be social whenever I can. It's easy for me to want to hole up, but I try to make dates with friends to grab coffee, go for a walk, or try new things. In fact, my most recent New Year's resolution was that every six to eight weeks, I would try something new with my friend Helen. So far we've taken a yoga class with rescued goats, hit the flea market at the Rose Bowl (an iconic LA tradition I'd never done before), hiked unfamiliar trails, and tried new restaurants. I also encourage our close friends to keep coming over to visit with Bruce. It's beautiful to see how they show up for him and all the love that surrounds him with his "core crew," as he called them.

## STAY ON TOP OF *YOUR* MEDICAL HEALTH

As I mentioned earlier in the book, for a while, I was super diligent about anything health-related for Bruce but put my own care on the back burner. I'm sure this sounds familiar to you, and if so, you're not alone.

"Regardless of how much they love their family members and want to support them in their illness, 23 percent of caregivers say doing so has made their own health worse," explains Dr. Sadeghi. "And not surprisingly, one study that found the highest death rates among caregivers revealed 45 percent skipped their own medical appointments because their caregiving did not allow the time."

It's taken a while, but now I make a conscious effort to take care of myself. For example, when I go for a checkup, I book the next mammogram or dental cleaning right then and there, even if it's six months or a year out. I also try to remind myself that it's not only okay if I have to put my needs above everyone else's, it's necessary.

I know you are busy caring for your loved one and monitoring their health, but it's crucial to stay on top of your own, too. Along these lines, it's important to know things like your blood pressure and cholesterol, as well as to monitor your sleep and exercise, which is pretty easy today since we have access to various trackers—many are on your phone. Again, let me say that if you're not prioritizing your own health and well-being, how can you fully care for someone else?


AS YOU KNOW by now, the focus of this entire book is that if you take better care of yourself, you can take better care of your person. Your brain health is a huge part of this because, let's face it, being a care partner requires a lot of thinking, planning, decision-making, and creativity. It takes brain power. As a result, if your cognitive function is not the best it can be, it just makes the hard job of being a care partner even harder. So while it's not always easy to implement these pillars of brain health, remember that all of them—exercise, good nutrition, sleep, stress reduction, and staying socially connected and on top of your medical health—go beyond your brain and help your whole body function better while boosting your physical and mental health. When I think of it that way, it motivates me to try to be my brain-healthy best. Also, if doing all of this at once is too overwhelming, pick one pillar to start with. Remember, it's never too late, and *something* is always better than nothing.

## Something to think about . . .

I realize that implementing the pillars of brain health can seem daunting when you are taking care of someone else. The first step is figuring out what's standing in your way. Dr. Lauren Massimo, associate professor of nursing at the University of Pennsylvania, whom we met in Chapter 4, suggests asking yourself about your barriers to doing these things and how you can reduce them. For example, why can't you get to bed before 1:00 a.m.? If helping with homework is the reason your night gets off track, see if your child's school offers some support.

To help you identify your barriers, answer the following questions and then reach out to a trusted friend, family member, therapist, or doctor to brainstorm ways to put these plans in place.

- What are my barriers to eating a brain-healthy diet?

_____

_____

_____

_____

_____

• How can I reduce those barriers to eating a brain-healthy diet?

_____

_____

_____

_____

_____

• What are my barriers to exercising?

_____

_____

_____

_____

_____

• How can I reduce those barriers to exercising?

_____

_____

_____

_____

_____

• What are my barriers to sleeping longer/more often?

_____

_____

_____

_____

_____

• How can I reduce those barriers to better sleep?

_____

_____

_____

_____

_____

• What are my barriers to implementing stress-reduction techniques?

_____

_____

_____

_____

_____

- How can I reduce those barriers so I can add stress-reduction techniques to my daily life?

_____

_____

_____

_____

_____

- What are my barriers to staying socially connected?

_____

_____

_____

_____

_____

- How can I reduce the barriers to staying socially connected?

_____

_____

_____

_____

_____

- What are my barriers to staying on top of my medical health?

_____

_____

_____

_____

_____

- How can I reduce the barriers to staying on top of my medical health?

_____

_____

_____

_____

_____

# SIX

# Expect an Array of Emotions

Much about caregiving is irritating, unattractive, and upsetting.
Expressing those feelings does not disrespect the loved one you're
caring for but validates your own suffering, sacrifice, and humanity in
the caregiving relationship. You have a right to your own emotional
process, and it's essential to engage it for your long-term well-being.

**HABIB SADEGHI,**
*DO, cofounder of Entelechy Medical Center*

To say my world has been rocked by Bruce's FTD is truly an understatement. We had our story written, our future mapped out. And yet all those hopes and dreams crumbled. That page in my notebook had to be torn out and tossed in the bin. And it wasn't just my life or Bruce's that changed. It was also the lives of our two young girls, who were ten and eight years old at the time of his diagnosis.

There were so many places that Bruce had traveled with his three older daughters that he couldn't wait to revisit with our younger ones. But Mabel and Evelyn won't get to share these special trips with their dad.

In addition, he won't be part of their big moments. He won't beam with pride at their graduations or dance with them or their older sisters at their weddings. And yet what really takes my breath away is the little stuff that they are missing out on. For example, Bruce would have loved

Evelyn's quick, sharp wit, and yet she won't get to banter with him and see how similar they are. And Mabel can turn anything into a piece of art, yet she's missing Bruce proudly displaying her creations on his office shelves or door along with a dozen others that he's already hung there. He was just that guy. The super-proud dad.

It's also mind-boggling to me that the parts of life that Bruce embraced with such energy and excitement won't happen again. Gone are the days when he tickled the girls until they squealed, especially during my calm and rigid bedtime routine. Gone are the days when he played with them in the pool and took them for ice cream.

For so long, Mabel and Evelyn thought I was out looking for a cure. After all, like most kids, their experience with illness has been that you get sick and then you get better. On top of this, they saw me throw everything and the kitchen sink at their father's disease because I didn't take well to his doctors saying, "There's nothing we can do." To prove them wrong and show my girls that I had not lost hope, I left no stone unturned, exploring different therapies that I was told could help Bruce. When nothing worked, I was devastated. Each and every time. Sharing the outcomes with the girls when they asked were some of the saddest, knife-in-my-heart moments.

Unfortunately, sadness isn't the only emotion I've experienced on this journey, and I'm sure you can relate. I cry a lot. I've screamed into my pillow. I've stomped my feet. Every emotion you can think of, I've had it. Plenty of times, this range of feelings has brought me to my knees. And I know you've been brought to your knees, too. Although no two dementia cases, care partners, or loved ones are the same, when I'm in a room with other caregivers and they talk about their feelings, it's a carbon copy of me to some degree.

What I wish I knew earlier was that a full spectrum of emotions comes with your person's diagnosis, and it's crucial to allow yourself to feel *all* of them.

## THE IMPORTANCE OF LETTING IT ALL OUT

"Suppressing emotions allows pressure to build up until it eventually explodes in a health or emotional crisis later on," explains Dr. Sadeghi. "As it's been said, feelings buried alive never die."

Adds my therapist, Kathleen Murphy, who specializes in helping people navigate relational and traumatic challenges: "It's like a teapot that has a top on and nowhere to express the excess steam. If you reach your capacity, you may behave in a way that you don't like; for example, exploding in anger at your person when they didn't really do anything. Then that turns into self-hatred and beating yourself up when most people in your situation would respond the same way."

The feelings are inevitable, so you'll want to practice embracing them without judgment. (There seems to be a lot of judgment on this journey!) For most care partners, this can be especially hard because our emotions are usually stuffed way down for several reasons.

First, the focus is on our person 24/7, and as we are trying to gain our footing, especially in the beginning, we don't have a chance to think about ourselves. This was the case with me. In those earlier days, I walked around barely connected to my own body.

Expressing our emotions is also considered to be a faux pas. Sometimes people who are not caregivers have a set view of what caregiving looks like and how you should be in this role. The perception is you're supposed to put your saint hat on and devote your whole life to your person without expressing anything other than sadness. Sharing other feelings may be viewed as complaining. I've heard people say, "How can *you* complain? What about the person this is happening to? Why don't you think about them?" Well, that's the thing: We are *always* thinking about them. Bruce is on my mind around the clock, whether I'm on a hike, at school drop-off, or sitting right next to him.

What I learned from my therapist, who was treating someone else whose husband had young-onset Alzheimer's, was that all my feelings and emotions were valid and reflected in her other patient, too. That was comforting because, at times, I felt guilt for feeling angry that life seemed so out of control, resentment that the future Bruce and I had envisioned was destroyed, dread that I'd be steering the entire ship of our lives alone, grief over all that we'd lost, and rage that I'd become a caregiver because my husband was sick. I just wanted him and our lives back.

What I now understand is while dementia might be playing out differently in our homes, the feelings and emotions we share as caregivers are very similar. So let's look at how they present themselves and how we can begin to recognize them.

## THERAPY

Before we get too far into this chapter, I want to talk briefly about what I feel is one of the best ways to handle your emotions and a tool you'll see me refer to frequently: therapy.

"The confidentiality of the therapeutic relationship allows you to talk about things that you don't feel safe talking about with anyone else," Kathleen explains. "Family and friends are often too close to your emotions to help you; a therapist doesn't bring any history or emotional baggage that may inhibit you being heard and seen."

Also, when it comes to caregiving, you are there for everyone else. A therapist is someone who is *just* there for you, and you don't have to worry about doing anything in return or feeling like a burden. Knowing that I can say whatever I want to my therapist without fear of judgment helps me express all my thoughts, which gets them out of my head and body and makes me feel lighter and less alone.

To find a therapist, ask your doctor, social worker, loved ones, or a close friend for recommendations. Group therapy can also help and may be less expensive. Thankfully, technology has made getting therapy a bit easier. Many therapists meet virtually, like on Zoom, so you don't have to leave home. If the fee is an issue, ask your therapist about a sliding scale—many offer these. Therapy apps and online therapy may be more affordable and, again, they make it easy to do without being too far from your person. Another option is to search for low-cost or free support groups or therapy at local hospitals, community centers, university health clinics, health centers, and nonprofit organizations. Your neurologist's office may have some insight on this, too.

## ANGER AND RESENTMENT

As I've mentioned, Bruce had always been my rock, and I felt safe and taken care of with him in my life. This feeling was a dream come true for me. So one of the harshest moments was realizing I no longer had a protector in him.

One night in the early days of Bruce seeming off, our house alarm blared at 2:00 a.m. I paused for a second, expecting Bruce to deal with it like he always did. But when he didn't even stir, I ran down the stairs from our bedroom and punched the code into the alarm keypad. In that moment it hit me, *Is this all on me now?* I was losing parts of Bruce slowly and it was just unbearable. I couldn't seem to make sense of it. So I dug my heels in and sat in anger and resentment. I was so pissed at him.

What Kathleen helped me do was turn my anger into something more productive, to reframe it as a natural and necessary reaction.

"We're taught that anger is bad but it's an emotion of protection," says Kathleen. This was certainly true for me: My anger served me. I'm not saying it was right or great for my health or frame of mind, but it did propel me forward. That energy allowed me to put one foot in front of the other. It made me determined to figure out: *What the hell is going on with my husband?*

Working with professionals like Kathleen and Dr. Sadeghi has allowed me the space to get it all out—the good, bad, and ugly—and process everything that's been lost. They don't tell me *how* to process, but they give me space to say out loud what I've been thinking, and they encourage me to talk openly and honestly about my anger and resentment without sugarcoating anything. They want me to be able to get it out, not keep it inside. That's what I tell my kids all the time: better out than in.

At first, this was so foreign to me. As I've mentioned, I tend to bottle up my emotions and soldier on, and I felt like Kathleen and Dr. Sadeghi would think I was a terrible person if I verbalized what I'd been keeping deep inside. *I'm sure no one else has these thoughts. I am the worst wife in the world. Am I really going to reveal this ugly side of me?* I took a leap of faith and am happy I did. I am better for it, especially as a care partner.

You need a space to be able to do this, too. Anger doesn't make you weak, selfish, or unkind. It makes you human. Caring for someone while holding so much inside is exhausting, and acknowledging the full range of your emotions is not only necessary, it's healthy. You are doing the best you can in an incredibly difficult situation, and giving yourself permission to feel it all is part of what makes you a compassionate and capable caregiver.

To process anger, resentment, and any of the other emotions discussed in this chapter, experts suggest joining support groups for dementia caregivers. There you'll find comfort in hearing others say "Me too" when you share your experience and emotions. Look for a support group at a church, community center, or memory care facility in your area. There are also support groups online. Or start your own, either by posting on social media or—the old-fashioned way—by hanging a sign up on a local bulletin board.

Other options you can consider are talking to a close, understanding, nonjudgmental friend, journaling, or therapy.

## WHEN YOU'RE ON YOUR OWN

You may not have someone to process your emotions with, and that's okay. Kathleen has shared some tips for doing so on your own:

- When you're feeling sad and upset, stop and put your hand on your heart. Take time to feel the actual sensation of your heart.

- Tell yourself, "Of course, I'm suffering. Anybody would be."

- Remind yourself that you're suffering because it's part of life, not because there's something wrong with you. You are human.

## FEAR

I've always been a fear-based person. You name it, I'm afraid of it. I'm afraid of flying. I'm afraid of speaking in public and saying the wrong thing. And then there are the bigger things that I don't even want to put into the atmosphere. I think it's because my parents' divorce showed me your life can be rocked in a split second. (It was not the news of their divorce that shook me; it was the aftereffect and how my life changed so drastically.) Throughout most of my adult life, my New Year's resolution has remained the same: to not let fear stop me.

Add this fear-based personality to the intense level of uncertainty I experienced as Bruce started to decline and the lack of control that

FTD gives you, and let's just say it felt like my fairy tale had turned into a living nightmare. I had many sleepless nights and a seemingly endless string of scary thoughts and worries swirling through my brain. I was distracted with a constant racing feeling inside my body.

Kathleen helped me normalize this reaction.

"Fear is the activation that there's danger, and if your loved one is not doing well, that's danger," she says. "The problem is when fear becomes constant."

I've had to work hard to shift myself from a state of constant fear into one of relative calm. One thing that's helped is the confidence I've built as a caregiver and manager of all the moving parts it entails. When I'm scared, I remind myself that I've been taking care of my husband and my two children in a difficult situation, and I know that I'm doing the best that I can. I'm capable and this is something to be proud of. I've come this far, and I know that when the next shoe drops, I will be able to figure it out. You have to be your own cheerleader, acknowledging each little win. I encourage you to consider creating similar affirmations for yourself to rely upon in moments of fear.

Another thing that's helped me combat my fear is becoming knowledgeable about Bruce's disease. I'm not afraid to ask questions, and I'm not afraid to hear the answers. I might not be able to change the situation, but I can change how I look at it and my feelings around it. As we discussed in Chapter 2, knowledge can help ground you when things feel uncertain and, as Teepa says, that's the key to reducing your stress. If you're that type of person, the next time you feel overwhelmed with fear, is there an expert you can reach out to for more information?

What I've also found is that most people in this community want to help because they connect with you in such a profound way; they want to provide resources and ideas to make things a little lighter for you. Since Bruce's diagnosis, several friends have had people in their lives newly diagnosed with young-onset dementia. When they reach out to me for resources, I'm always happy to help. And maybe that's a given, as I'm writing a book to share what I know with you.

Kathleen also taught me the following steps to help calm my nervous system when I'm afraid, so I can begin to see things differently. I'm hoping they will help you so that fear doesn't control your world as much anymore:

1. Recognize that you are in fear. Tell yourself, "I'm in fear."

2. Give yourself compassion and breathe.

3. Ask yourself, "Am I in danger? Is my loved one in danger?" Most of the time you will realize the fear is just a habitual response and you are actually safe.

4. Use a calm internal voice and talk to yourself like you would a child. Rather than beat yourself up, say things like, "I know you're scared. It's all right. You're safe right now. There's nothing to fear in this moment."

5. Soften your eye gaze. When you're scared, your gaze gets intense, and your eyes widen. Softening them seems to activate your nervous system in ways that help you feel safe and calm.

6. Fold your arms across your chest and use your hands to stroke or pat your upper arms the way you would touch a child to soothe them. At the same time, use that soft internal voice to say, "It's okay. We got this. Yes, you wish things were different, but here we are."

All of this might sound far-fetched or maybe even silly, but it's so important to acknowledge your suffering and to be kind to yourself.

## GRIEF

In 2024 I was asked to attend the International Conference on Fronto-temporal Dementias (ISFTD) in Amsterdam, which brought together people who are making a difference within the FTD world. There, I was able to give some remarks to 750 researchers and scientists, participate in a panel discussion, join a day designed for caregivers and people living with FTD, and just be a fly on the wall to hear about potential new developments in treatment. The Association for Frontotemporal Degeneration (AFTD) had their own room in the same building as the conference and told me I could use it if I needed to take a breather at any point.

One afternoon, I was in that room collecting myself when Tracey Wardill, MA, PhD, a clinical neuropsychologist and director of Neuropsychology Melbourne, came in. I'd met Tracey the first day of the conference.

"How are you doing?" she asked, knowing how intense four days focusing on FTD must be for me as a care partner. That's when I broke down. During the conference, I tried to be so buttoned-up and professional, and despite getting choked up when speaking on a panel and giving my remarks, I'd held it together for days. But in that moment, I had reached a limit, and I had a full-blown cry.

"It's just so hard," I said. Those were the only words I could manage in between giant sobs.

"Emma, I understand," Tracey said with tears in her eyes. "Let's just sit here and cry together." In that moment, that was exactly what I needed. The truth is, there's nothing anyone can do, say, or fix. And I'm grateful that Tracey was at the receiving end of it. She allowed me the space to just be and grieve. This act was so loving and compassionate.

I didn't even realize how scary grief could be and how uncomfortable it could make me until I was talking to Patti Davis, the friend and mentor we met earlier whose father was President Reagan. She reminded me that "grief constantly asks us to acknowledge it, but most of us want to avoid it because it hurts and it's scary. Alzheimer's offers ample opportunities for avoidance because you have so many hands-on caregiving duties that you have no time to even think about grief."

When Patti said this, I had a realization. I thought about all the things I do to keep myself ultra-busy so that I don't have to feel it. For example, for so long, my quest to understand Bruce's diagnosis kept me hungry for answers and laser-focused on how best to support my family. And being pissed off and resentful allowed me to push those immense feelings of grief to the side because if I really took the time and felt them, I don't know how I would be able to function.

Patti taught me that it's important to acknowledge your grief early on. When someone new came to the support groups that she ran, first at UCLA Medical Center and then at Saint John's in Santa Monica, California, she would always ask, "How are you doing with your grief?" She told me that some people would answer, but others would look at her like she was crazy because their person was still alive.

"Why would I be grieving?" they'd ask her.

She explained to me how she'd answer.

"I'd tell them, this disease is sort of a death before dying. You're losing a lot so the grieving process really needs to start now. Yes, it's scary. It's like crossing this river and there are currents underneath. Sometimes you feel like you're being pulled under and think you're going to drown. But you *will* get to the other side. And you'll be different when you get there. It just takes a lot of faith, and it takes a decision to sit with your grief."

So how do you do that? How do you sit with your grief?

The first step is to acknowledge it. Tell yourself, *I'm grieving.* Sometimes we don't realize what we're feeling until we put a name to it.

The second is to give yourself space and time to grieve. It's okay to cry and mourn what was and what could have been. It's okay to be sad about what this disease has taken from your loved one and you. The feeling is relentless, and you need those moments to break down. This is one reason why caregivers often have no tears left when their loved one eventually passes away. People in their lives don't realize how much they've cried and grieved along the way already.

The third is realizing that grief is not linear. Prior to becoming a care partner, I'd heard about the five stages of grief; however, I'm not sure this makes sense with a disease like FTD. And yes, I understand that the five stages are supposed to apply to someone who has passed, but this is dementia we are talking about. We grieve while our person is still alive. To me, the five stages imply that you go through each stage and then you are done. In my experience so far with grief, the intensity you feel might decrease over time, but it's not as if one day you're grieving and then you're not grieving. It's more like waves in the ocean, which ebb and flow. Sometimes those waves are huge, sometimes they are subtle. I teeter between grief and trauma. It all depends on the day.

The fourth is to recognize that you are adaptable, and while your grief may change over time, you will become stronger because of it. Recently, I was talking to a friend of mine and Bruce's about his disease. I hadn't seen her in a while, so I was giving her the update. As I did, tears streamed down her face. I totally understood her feelings. After all, I'm an empath, so it doesn't take much to bring tears to my eyes. But I didn't cry with her. Over time I have built up strength and have adapted to this "new norm." I later learned that this is what Tali Sharot, director of the Affective Brain Lab in London, calls emotional habituation.

"Studies show that the feelings associated with loss subside over time. Sometimes it's slow, but we habituate and adapt," says Sharot. "This doesn't mean we don't care or suffer, but our physiological and affective reaction is reduced."

I never thought this would happen to me, but I have habituated to Bruce and his disease and to the grief and sadness surrounding it. It is such a part of my daily life and takes up so much space in my head that it's my new normal. In the early days, I was flooded with emotions when I talked about this turn our lives have taken, but today I don't break down as frequently, and now I understand why. The positive side of this effect is that now I can be there for friends and family when they want to grieve about what's being taken away from *them*. I can let them have their feelings and be a strong shoulder for them to cry on. Or there are days when I can be like Tracey and just cry alongside them.

The last thing I like to remind myself is a quote my stepdaughter Scout shared with me: "Grief is the price we pay for loving someone so deeply." Grief is painful, but that pain reflects the love and special connection you had, and still have, with someone who means everything to you. In that way, grief can be seen as a continuation of love, a way to stay connected to them and honor your relationship. For me, the grief I feel over what's happening is rooted in the deep love I have for Bruce and my family. There is so much beauty in that. And here's the truth: No one in this world will escape grief—it's a universal part of loving and living.

Some resources to help you process your grief, as with other emotions, are support groups, therapy, and friends. You also might want to check out the workbook put out by AFTD called *Walking with Grief: Loss and the FTD Journey*, which you can find on their website.

## EMPATHIC DISTRESS

Empathy is an important part of being a care partner to someone with dementia. Since in many cases you can't rely on your person to clearly express how they're feeling, you must be his or her eyes and ears. I can't go to Bruce and ask him what's wrong. I have to look at him and read his body language. However, if you're overly empathetic like me, you can take on too much internally, a phenomenon called empathic distress.

"Empathic distress is feeling distressed because you're overidentifying and projecting what your loved one must feel like," Kathleen explains. "It's imagining that, *If I were Bruce, I would feel this way* because you're seeing him as having the same brain as you and the same experience as you. So you're thinking, *He might be lonely*, and then that breaks your heart. And yet that isn't his experience."

As caregivers, we have to protect ourselves from over-caring because this level of added stress is a recipe for more sadness and grief and can make you physically sick and prevent you from being the best care partner you can be. I tend to take residence in Bruce's head, projecting my own feelings onto the situation. For my own health, I've had to learn how to separate myself from Bruce's experience. I haven't perfected this, but when I find myself engaging in empathic distress, I take a moment to comfort myself and acknowledge that, yes, this is hard, and I hate this for him, but then I take a minute to get out of Bruce's body and back into my own. I know this might sound wild, but I visualize myself in a bubble (it acts as a shield), which allows me to really look at Bruce and tend to him in a way that isn't clouded by my own perception that sometimes is just not accurate. As Dr. Sadeghi always tells me, "This is hard stuff, black-belt stuff that you are doing."

When you find yourself in these moments, remind yourself: *What I am witnessing and going through is incredibly difficult. It's okay to feel that.* Acknowledging this doesn't mean you are stepping away from your person, it means you are stepping into the clarity needed to support them in the best way possible.

I also tell myself, "Stay here, don't go there."

"'Stay here, don't go there' is about not getting into other people's heads," Kathleen explains. "It's an internal boundary where you don't allow yourself to imagine a scenario that creates unnecessary suffering." Yes, we want to have empathy for others, it's a trait that's an important part of being human. But when it comes to caregiving, we need to figure out how to skillfully use our empathy to care while also stepping back and noticing that our loved ones are *not* feeling what we're feeling, and they are not thinking what we're thinking. Practice creating emotional boundaries by staying here, not going there.

Over time, sitting in constant empathic distress serves no one. In fact, it can even lead to trauma, which we'll address more later in the chapter.

"If you're in a constant state of trauma, you're no longer able to read your environment accurately, so you can't trust your intuition and might see danger where there isn't any," explains Kathleen. This makes it harder to access or even recognize the resources available, and ultimately you start to lose trust in your decisions and stop feeling safe in the world.

"Connection with others can aid in healing trauma because it helps to restore your nervous system so that you can be calm enough to have confidence in your decisions and feel safe," says Kathleen. Again, a support group or finding just one other person in your caregiving dementia shoes can help bring the volume down a little bit.

---

"While embracing and expressing your emotions is important, it's equally important that you don't do so in the presence of the person you're caring for. This process is a private one and you don't want your loved one to feel personally responsible for upsetting you. They didn't plan to get sick and, depending on where they are in their disease, may already feel bad that they have to ask for your help."

**DR. HABIB SADEGHI,**
*cofounder of Entelechy Medical Center*

---

## GUILT

There's so much guilt that comes with being a caregiver. For me, it was and still can be a pervasive feeling, creeping in and visiting me daily. Guilt about feeling frustrated. Guilt about being resentful at the turn our lives have taken. Guilt about not having understood the early signs of Bruce's disease. Guilt around not being the best caregiver I can be, and guilt about not being the best mom I can be. Guilt that there are times I hate having to be a caregiver. Then there's guilt that I've hired professional caregivers, and guilt that I have resources to do so when so many others don't. Oh, and then there's the guilt when I do something Bruce and I dreamed of doing with our girls but he can't come, and even guilt about just having fun. And this happens even with all the work I've done on myself. It's nonstop. But as dementia specialist Teepa Snow says, "Not carrying around guilt is super vital for care partners because feeling guilty just distracts you from care and life."

"Guilt is actually a normal part of being a care partner. In fact, if you didn't feel guilt, it wouldn't be normal. It's how you process the guilt that matters," explains Arlene Schollaert, family services director of Amazing Place in Houston, Texas.

So what do you do with all that guilt?

First, give yourself the opportunity to say it out loud and process it, whether that's in a support group or with a counselor or a therapist. This is important because guilt can be a roadblock to caring for yourself. (This was the case with me, as we talked about in Chapter 4.)

When I'm dealing with guilt, sometimes the best thing I can do is think about that scene in *Moonstruck* when Cher slaps Nicolas Cage and says, "Snap out of it!" My version is telling myself, *Get a grip, Emma*, to bring me back to what is true: that I am taking care of my husband and family to the best of my ability. I wasn't trained for this! I'm learning new skills in real time so there needs to be room for error. I will go to my grave knowing I did all that I possibly could with the tools and resources I was given. Of course, I have not done it all perfectly, but I have grown from this experience. I will continue to put my best foot forward.

Find your own Cher line (or use mine) to bring yourself back when you're feeling guilty and then follow it up with what you know in your heart to be true: You are doing the best you can in what are incomprehensible circumstances.

## CONFUSION/AMBIGUITY

FTD doesn't scream. It whispers. And it does so for so long that it's unclear that your loved one is slipping away. We had been losing Bruce slowly and we didn't know it. And even when I suspected something was wrong, I never fathomed it would be a form of dementia. Bruce was too young for that, or so I thought, and I'd never heard of young-onset dementia. It just wasn't on my radar.

Thinking back on the timeline of Bruce's disease, it's hard to know when and where it began to rear its ugly head. Early-onset dementia is insidious, sneaking in slowly and subtly altering the person you've always known, making slight changes until the person you love feels like a distant version of who they once were. This gray area is hard for me because I sometimes think, *When was the last time I had* all *of Bruce? What were we doing? What was that last conversation I had with him?* Unfortunately, I will never know the answers to those questions, and yet that still eats away at me. This is part of something called ambiguous loss.

Dr. Pauline Boss, a professor emeritus at the University of Minnesota, has done groundbreaking research on the theory of ambiguous loss. She was also a caregiver to her husband, so she knows firsthand what ambiguous loss feels like.

"Ambiguous loss is an unclear loss," she explains. "It can be about a person who is physically absent but psychologically present. For example, kidnapped children or soldiers missing in action. Or it can be when the person is physically present but psychologically absent due to some illness or condition, such as dementia."

The idea of ambiguous loss was something I had never heard of before. But as I went down the learning-about-dementia road, it was a term that came up time and time again. I can guarantee that now that you are on this journey, you will hear it a lot, too, because ambiguous loss and dementia go hand in hand. When I learned about it, I was struck by how perfectly it defined what I was experiencing. In Chapter 1, I shared all the things I loved about Bruce in the past tense, even though he's still right in front of me. Of course, I still love so much about him as he is today, but those things that disappeared without me realizing are at the core of ambiguous loss: The person is right in front of you, but they don't represent who they were.

Ambiguous loss is immensely painful and not well understood by other people unless they've gone through it. In fact, in my experience, people can be very judgmental because they don't understand what it is or what it feels like to know or love someone with dementia. For example, if I say that I feel grief, it's usually met with some form of "Why? Bruce is still here," or "How could you be grieving someone who is still alive?" or "You should feel lucky you still have him." But learning about this phenomenon reassured me that this loss is a real feeling. I hope you find comfort in the fact that there's a name for this kind of loss, it's real, and you're not alone.

## TRAUMA

Although trauma might not be an emotion, it *is* an emotional response to difficult events that can bring up fear, anger, loss, and sadness, among many other feelings, so I'd like to talk about it here. Even with all the work I've done, trauma still sits right at the surface for me, and it's one part of this experience that I know I need to address.

Watching Bruce change has been nothing short of devastating. Seeing our children witness it, while having a front-row seat to the toll it's taken on them, has been a hard pill to swallow. I've come to realize that I'm far from processing the full extent of this trauma. And as I think about Bruce's progression, I often ask myself: How will I cope? These are the moments when I have to remind myself, "Stay here. Don't go there," which not only helps with empathic distress, but is also a reminder about remaining in the present and not borrowing tomorrow's worries.

When I attended the ISFTD conference in Amsterdam, I went to a presentation given by Katie Brandt of the Frontotemporal Disorders Unit at Massachusetts General Hospital, who had been a caregiver for her husband before he passed away from FTD. Her goal was to offer fresh insights to help caregivers prepare for the road ahead, equipping them without overwhelming them. As I sat in the back of the room, tears streamed down my face. I was flooded with memories of being a new caregiver, starting at square one, just like the care partners in that room. I watched them hang on to her every word, scribbling notes and absorbing every bit of Katie's wisdom. I was transported back to how hopeless and lost I felt in those early days.

The emotions in that room were overwhelming. These new caregivers were already grappling with the confusion and frustration that FTD brings, now realizing they had to dive in headfirst. There's no halfway with this disease, it demands everything. I left the room feeling one step away from a panic attack. That was the end of the conference for me; I couldn't stay another minute. For the sake of my own well-being, I had to leave.

Lately, I've been doing more advocacy work that involves speaking engagements, and there's one part of my remarks that I struggle to get through without crying. It's when I share the moment we received our diagnosis. (I say "our" because FTD, or any form of dementia, is a family disease.) I talk about how we were told, "There's nothing we can do," and were sent away with a pamphlet and not a single resource. I end my remarks with this line:

"I hold on to the belief that one day soon, families like mine won't have to hear 'There's nothing we can do.' Instead, they'll hear: 'We have treatments that will help, and a road map to guide you in your new role.'"

I've never been able to say that line without crying. The news we received in the doctor's office that day, *There is nothing that can be done*, was the worst of my life. And leaving with no direction was just as bad. It has left a lasting imprint of trauma on me.

While I'm okay with showing emotion, I recognize that this moment strikes a deep chord in me, one I haven't fully processed.

It could be anger, frustration, or trauma. Probably all of the above. I know advocacy, empowering the next caregiver, and raising awareness are vital to me, but I also need to remember that I'm human. If I want to sustain this work with the intensity it requires and keep showing up, I need to address my trauma.

Recently, a colleague suggested that I work with a trauma coach. Her advice has stayed with me: If I haven't processed the trauma from the beginning of this journey, how will I manage as more unfolds? Sometimes we need this gentle push to open our eyes.

For any care partner reading this, please do yourself a favor: Start acknowledging your emotions. Allow yourself to feel them and find ways to process them. These feelings won't go away, and we can't avoid them, but we can't afford to sit in the unprocessed versions of them either. It's not healthy. Seek out support, whether through a therapist, a trauma coach, or another trusted resource I have given you in this chapter.

We can't control the trauma this disease brings, but we can control how we take care of ourselves through it.

## HOW TO MANAGE ALL YOUR EMOTIONS

We must remember that this journey is long; dementia usually progresses slowly, so we need to develop coping strategies that will help us process all the emotions we will feel over time. When I allow myself to do this, I'm stronger and my energy is better. Instead of bringing unprocessed guilt and sadness into the room with Bruce—and trust me, your loved one feels your energy—I use the tools we've discussed so far: therapy, talking with a friend, mantras, self-calming, and meditation. Here are two other tools I've found to be invaluable. I hope they help you, too.

### *Purge Emotional Writing*

I'm still on this journey of grief and have immense sadness in my heart, but I have come a long, long way. Of course, I have moments when I cry and even scream. But I'm happy to report that being allowed the space to get out and process those feelings has helped me so much.

One of the ways I do this is when a feeling of grief, anger, or resentment arises, I write it down on a piece of paper. I learned this form of self-therapy from Dr. Sadeghi. It's called Purge Emotional Writing, or PEW-12.

"It's an exercise I give all my patients who need to release stress from unresolved emotional issues," says Dr. Sadeghi. By consistently doing this, over time, you're drawing the poison energy out and making room for healing energy to replace it. What follows is his exercise and insight:

- Get some paper and a pen and find a quiet place to sit. This exercise doesn't work on a computer or any electronic device. The physical energetic connection is important, and that only comes from doing it in your own handwriting.

- Set a timer for ten to twelve minutes.

- Start writing in a stream-of-consciousness manner about whatever is on your mind—caregiving, finances, work, relationships, etc.—and don't stop to edit or worry about spelling, grammar, handwriting, or anything else. This exercise works best if you just keep on writing and let the feelings flow.

- This is not the time to be polite. Write whatever you want—no one else is going to see it.

- You may get to the point where your emotions are flowing so quickly that you can't even write real words anymore. That's fine. It doesn't need to be legible, and it means that the fire is really flowing. Just maintain contact between the pen and paper.

- When the timer goes off, stop writing.

- Do not reread what you've written. (This can reinfect you with the negative energy.)

- Immediately take the pages to a fire-safe and secure place, such as a fireplace or grill, and set them ablaze.

Fire is particularly cleansing and transformational. Your goal is to neutralize the negative energy, and fire does that by changing the chemical composition of the paper to ash. However, destroying the pages in another safe way—like in a paper shredder or just ripping them up—works, too. (I've actually never set them on fire because it makes me nervous.)

- Do this several times a week until you feel the emotional shift as your burden of negative energy becomes lighter and lighter.

### Give Yourself Thirty

This is something Patti Davis taught me that I really love. Whenever you experience a messy emotion, remind yourself that you are allowed to have that emotion, but set a time limit on it. For example, if you're angry, set a timer on your phone for thirty minutes and allow yourself to be pissed off for thirty minutes. Tell yourself, "This is how I'm feeling now, but after thirty minutes, I'm going to remember how to be at peace." Decide that once that timer goes off, you're done. There's no wiggle room; you can't hit the snooze button.

"I would never tell you not to feel something. But I would have you ask yourself if that's where you want to live," says Patti. Remember: You have a choice not to live in those emotions and to move on.

AS YOU FINISH this chapter, please remember: All your emotions are valid. Most care partners have them even if you haven't heard anyone else express them. (And if you haven't, this is why it's so important to connect with and find a community, because that is where you *will* hear others say out loud what you've been silently thinking.) It's important to try to process this roller coaster of emotions in any and all ways, and to remember you're not alone.

## QUESTIONS AND ANSWERS WITH DR. PAULINE BOSS

Dr. Pauline Boss is the author of six books that have been so helpful to me, especially *Loving Someone Who Has Dementia: How to Find Hope While Coping with Stress and Grief*, and I've learned so much from talking to her, especially about ambiguous loss. Here Dr. Boss, who was a caregiver for her husband, talks more about this term that she coined.

**People can be very judgmental about this idea of ambiguous loss. Usually it's met with "But this person is still in front of you. Why or how could you be grieving someone who is still alive?"**

Such people are thinking only about grief after death, but this is a situation where somebody *gradually* fades away. What you have is a loss that is not definitive. There's no finality to it. It's just each day, week, or month, you notice you've lost something new. For example, you can't travel together anymore, and then as time goes on, this person may not even know who you are, or as time goes on further, they may not even be able to swallow. It's very hard to find hope and meaning during this time. What I'm trying to do is to give this kind of loss a name so that people don't think they're going crazy, because it is a very, very confusing kind of loss with the person still physically present but psychologically absent.

The grief that comes from this is a frozen grief. It's not like the grief at a funeral home with a death certificate and a body to bury. It's a confusing grief because the person has not died. And yet there is much to grieve: the things you did together, the happy times you shared, the support you had. All of that is gone.

### How do we deal with frozen grief?

One of the tools that I recommend is "both/and" thinking. This is not typical of Americans who usually prefer linear thinking and certainty. This dialectical way of thinking is a more Eastern way of seeing a situation where you consider multiple perspectives. For example, you say to yourself, "Bruce is *both* here *and* he is also gone." This is as close to the truth as you can get since you have a partial thing to grieve—what you've lost about your person—and a partial thing to be happy about—that he's still here and you can still touch him. The stress of living with ambiguity and ambiguous loss is huge, so you have to manage it in a way that you can continue to function. "Both/and" thinking is a useful way to do that in your very challenging life as a caregiver.

### How can care partners thrive while living with ambiguous loss?

For many people, it's going to go on a long time, so you have to stay strong in order to bear it. You need to embrace the ambiguity because it's not going to go away. So that "both/and" thinking really helps. "He's here" and "he's also not here." That's really hard for us to do, but it can be learned. Don't let anyone tell you absolutes because neither one of those absolutes is correct. It's both/and. It's terrible AND yet something in your life is wonderful. For example, a caregiver might say, "I have a terrible loss. And I also have wonderful kids and he helped give them to me." Thinking in that way may lighten the load a bit.

**What are your thoughts on acceptance?**

I'm not terribly fond of the word "acceptance" because it means you have to surrender. I prefer you say, "I've decided to accept," which means *you* have more agency because it was your decision. In general, caregivers have trouble with agency because you are caught in a situation outside of your control. And most of us, at least in Western cultures, like to be in charge of our own day and destiny. As caregivers, we aren't in charge so we have to find something we can control in each day, even if it's small.

For example, during the COVID pandemic, when people felt so out of control with this ambiguous virus that we didn't know anything about, they were baking bread. Why? It gave them something to control for a couple of hours and it had a very nice outcome. That was really smart. Other people find agency in other ways—exercising or playing an instrument—something you can control. You need a little bit of that every day to balance the situation of ambiguous loss. That's true for all caregivers. It also helps to think about some new hope and purpose because having no agency and no hope is too much to bear. Balance it with some new hope, meaning, and purpose.

## *Something to think about . . .*

What are some of the emotions you've experienced on this journey?

_____

_____

_____

_____

_____

_____

_____

_____

_____

_____

_____

_____

_____

_____

_____

_____

_____

_____

_____

_____

# SEVEN

# Parenting While Caregiving

When you have children on this journey,
it's a diagnosis of the family.

**DIANA SHULLA COSE,**
*founding executive director of*
*Lorenzo's House*

They say parenting is one of the hardest jobs in the world. Well, so is caregiving. Combine the two, and the world's hardest jobs start to seem downright impossible. What makes this dual work even more unique is that the game is always changing. Your kids are growing, so their needs constantly shift, and as your loved one's disease progresses, his or her needs change, too. And if your partner is the one with dementia and is therefore increasingly unable to share in parenting responsibilities, life can feel truly overwhelming. At least, that's how it felt for me.

When I first sensed things were shifting and not feeling right with Bruce, Mabel and Evelyn were still very young, so I kept the details to myself. However, as they got older, I shared just enough information. For example, when Bruce's language and processing were affected, I told them, "This means that your dad may not fully understand what you're saying." (Even before this, I've always been direct with my kids. When they were babies, I spoke to them in full sentences as I've never been a fan of baby talk or oversimplifying things.) They were too young to understand the gravity of the situation, but they could understand that Bruce was losing an important communication skill. As their vocabulary was expanding, Bruce's was decreasing. I didn't want them to think that their dad didn't care about what they had to say just because he might not be able to respond appropriately, or that what was occurring was his fault or done on purpose. At the time, I also knew that a diagnosis was imminent, and sharing this small piece of information in advance felt better than dropping a big diagnosis on them out of nowhere.

When we finally found out that Bruce had FTD with PPA, Mabel was ten and Evelyn was eight. I told them the name of the disease and described what it meant and how it explained the symptoms Bruce had been displaying. They didn't have many questions. In fact, I believe they felt a sense of relief. Bruce's disease was no longer something abstract; we now had a name for it. Struggling to pronounce "frontotemporal dementia" and unable to remember the order of the letters FTD, the girls came up with an acronym that would help them: Fantastic Turtles Dancing. We couldn't help but smile and chuckle envisioning these fantastic turtles dancing in Bruce's head.

Of course, this is still painful for them on many levels, especially when your father is Bruce Willis and there are fabricated tabloid headlines like "The Family's Last Goodbye" or "The Family Doesn't Know If Bruce Will Make It to the Holidays." The way some media outlets have incorrectly framed his FTD diagnosis has only stigmatized dementia further.

These outlets have had countless opportunities to shift the narrative—to educate, foster compassion, and deepen understanding—but time and again, they miss the mark. It's clear they haven't done their homework, or perhaps they're simply fortunate that dementia hasn't touched their own families.

Initially, it hurt me to hear these made-up clickbait stories, and I didn't want the girls to be blindsided by them. Especially walking through the grocery store and seeing their dad on the cover of a tabloid, paired with some outlandish headline.

I also never knew what other children might say about Bruce on the playground because they heard their parents talking. Now my girls have the proper language to address another child's comment or question. (Even I have my own banked responses to pull from!) I've made it clear that they could come to me with any and all information. "If you hear anything that's confusing or makes you feel uneasy, always ask me," I said.

One person who has made it easier for me to walk our girls through this slow and difficult experience is Megan Graham, MS, CCLS. Megan is the vice president of research operations at Private Health Management, a company I consulted to help navigate the complicated medical landscape of dementia and make sure no stone was left unturned in terms of Bruce's care, treatments, and trials he could participate in. Megan has a background in providing emotional support to hospitalized children and those with ill parents. Her brilliant insight has been invaluable in helping me help my girls.

For this chapter, I asked Megan and a few other experts who have helped me about the most crucial things parents need to know as they navigate the dual roles of caregiving and parenting. Whether you're helping your child understand a parent's diagnosis of young-onset dementia or a grandparent's diagnosis of dementia (or even other illnesses), her insights will be valuable in navigating next steps. I think doing so helps make your life as a parent more manageable, too. There's that expression that "you are only as happy as your unhappiest child," which I find to be true. When our kids are struggling, it weighs on us deeply. But when we know they are cared for and supported, even during tough times, we can move through life with a little more ease.

## HOW TO HAVE THE CONVERSATION

I know I can't control the pain of this experience for my daughters, but what I *can* control is our conversations around their dad's disease. You can do this, too. By having the right support in place and learning the best way to communicate, we can help our children navigate and adapt to a situation that is constantly changing, and hopefully lower some of their anxiety in the process.

### Give Just Enough Info

The way you share a diagnosis with your child will depend on their age and development. For example, you would explain FTD to a four-year-old differently than you would a seventeen-year-old.

"What stays the same is that we're including the kids in the conversation, no matter their age," says Megan.

Megan was the one who told me to give Mabel and Evelyn some information but not more than they needed, since this kind of news can be overwhelming. (After all, I know how overwhelming it was for me, so I can't imagine what it would be like for a child.) And no one knows your child and what level of information they can handle better than you. For me, this included telling them the name of the disease— "Daddy has frontotemporal dementia, which some people refer to as FTD"—and then briefly explaining what that meant. After that, I provided information based off the questions they asked.

This can work for you, too. Determine how much information your child needs without overwhelming them. Megan suggests sharing it in digestible pieces. For example, "Right now, the doctors are focusing on helping Mom deal with her pain," instead of "Mom is really sick, and we don't know what's going to happen." The latter can create unnecessary fear and uncertainty. Instead, framing the information in a way that provides reassurance and stability helps children process things in a more manageable way. Then build on that according to their questions. And when you answer them, do so honestly, which doesn't mean you have to tell them all the details, or that you need to know all the information—it just means not telling them a lie.

That said, don't get too far ahead of the disease unless they ask. For example, if your child says, "Will Mommy need surgery?" be up-front and clear but don't get into whether the disease is terminal or if treatment is needed after the surgery, unless they inquire about this. Then pay attention to their reactions.

"Every child processes stress in their own way, and their struggles may not always be immediately apparent, but being aware of the different ways children might be struggling can help parents provide necessary support," says Danielle Cornacchio, PhD, a clinical child psychologist and director of the WaveMind Clinic and another person who has helped me navigate this journey with my girls.

Normal grief and stress reactions may include not feeling well. For example, they have stomachaches or don't want to go to school. It may also mean that they temporarily regress when it comes to certain behaviors. For example, those who are potty-trained may wet the bed, those who are independent may become clingy or may start throwing tantrums again. "These are normal reactions and typically temporary," says Megan.

On the flip side, "a child may need additional support outside of their family and friends, if their emotions and behaviors are impacting their daily activities or relationships," says Danielle. For example, you have a kid who loves playing soccer and suddenly they don't want to be on the team. Or you have a really social child who doesn't want to have playdates and sleepovers anymore. Other concerns are a significant change in their grades or prolonged fluctuations in their sleep, mood, and eating habits. If you notice these signs, it can help to get your child some extra support. Speak to his or her pediatrician and see if bringing in some form of therapy might be a good idea.

"Professional support, such as therapy, can provide children with coping strategies, and can also equip parents with tools to support their child through this difficult time," says Danielle.

Explain that often kids and adults will see a therapist to help them through challenging situations. This way therapy seems like a tool, not a punishment. You can say, "It can help to talk to an adult besides your parents or someone you know about your feelings. Would you like to meet someone who helps kids your age with things like this?"

## GUIDANCE BY AGE GROUP

Although each child is different, Megan offers age-appropriate best practices for communicating with your child:

### AGE 5-9 (EARLY SCHOOL AGE):

- **Capacity:** Concrete thinkers who benefit from simple, honest explanations.

- **Approach:** Use clear, age-appropriate language: "Mommy is very sick, and the doctors are doing everything they can to help her feel better." Avoid euphemisms that can confuse them, like "Daddy is feeling under the weather," which could minimize the seriousness of an illness and confuse the child when Daddy doesn't recover like he would from a cold.

- **Focus:** Reassure them of their safety and routine. Explain how their lives may change but emphasize that their needs will still be met.

### AGE 10-13 (MIDDLE SCHOOL AGE):

- **Capacity:** More capable of understanding the concept of illness and its impact. May begin to worry about death but still need reassurance.

- **Approach:** Provide slightly more detailed explanations, including the possibility of worsening health, while highlighting efforts to manage it. Encourage them to ask questions. For example, "Grandma has an illness that is affecting how her brain works. That's why she might have trouble remembering things, get confused, or act differently than she used to. The doctors are helping us manage her symptoms, but this type of illness changes over time. If you ever have questions or feelings about it, you can always talk to me—we'll figure it out together."

- **Focus:** Acknowledge their emotional reactions and normalize them. Offer opportunities for involvement, such as helping with caregiving in small, age-appropriate ways.

## AGE 14 AND UP:

- **Capacity:** Able to grasp abstract concepts and long-term implications. May grapple with existential concerns and emotional intensity.

- **Approach:** Share honest, comprehensive information. For instance, "I want to be honest with you about what's happening. Grandpa has a disease called Alzheimer's that's affecting his brain, which means over time, he may have more trouble remembering things, understanding conversations, or recognizing people. We don't know exactly how things will change, but we're doing everything we

can to make sure he's comfortable and supported.
If you ever want to talk or ask questions—I'm
here for you. You are not going through this alone,
and however you feel about it is completely okay."
Allow your children to process emotions at their
own pace and express them in their preferred way.
For example, do they like to talk or prefer to write
in a journal, paint, or draw?

- **Focus:** Offer opportunities for autonomy, like
choosing which family events to attend or deciding
how to share updates with friends. Validate their
feelings without rushing them to "move on." Also,
this age group may have a heightened need for independence and privacy. Respect their boundaries
but remain available for discussions.

## Be Truthful

We always want to protect our kids, but what I learned is the importance of being honest all along the journey.

"Kids know something is going on even if you're not telling them,
and if we don't talk about a diagnosis openly, they'll use what we call
'magical thinking' to create their own scenarios," Megan explains.
"Those scenarios are often a lot scarier than what's actually going on,
and they're not grounded in reality."

This is why we need to own these conversations with our children.

It may seem strange to share information with our kids that seems scary or overwhelming because we don't want to worry or upset them further. "However, when they feel included in the conversation, their anxiety decreases, making it easier for them to cope with the diagnosis," says Megan. This also helps them see that it's okay to ask questions and that they will get honest answers. They will also feel heard, which helps validate their emotions.

While you should be honest with your kids, also be mindful about discussing your loved one's diagnosis when kids are within earshot. Sometimes I talk about Bruce to another adult when the kids are in the room. I learned not to share anything in those moments that Mabel and Evelyn don't already know, even if it seems like they are not paying attention. Kids pick up a lot more than we think.

## WHAT TO SAY?

Talking to children about a loved one's dementia can feel overwhelming, but simple, honest language can help them process what's happening. Below are examples of what you might say to acknowledge their emotions, involve them in care, and prepare them for changes, depending on their age and understanding.

### ACKNOWLEDGE EMOTIONS:

- **Younger children:** "It's okay to feel sad, mad, or confused about what's happening. I feel that way sometimes, too."

- **Older children and teens:** "We can talk anytime you're feeling upset or have questions."

## INVOLVE THEM IN CARE:

- **Younger children:** "You can help by sitting with Dad and showing him your drawings."

- **Older children and teens:** "Would you like to help me make a playlist of Mom's favorite songs?"

## PREPARE FOR BEHAVIORAL CHANGES:

- **All ages:** "Sometimes Dad might say things that don't make sense or seem angry for no reason. It's not because of you—it's just the way the illness works."

## ENCOURAGE CONNECTION:

- **All ages:** "Even though Mom might not always seem like herself, she still loves spending time with you. Let's find activities you both enjoy, like puzzles, watching movies, or looking through old photos."

- Note that with FTD or other forms of dementia, sometimes there just might not be things that keep that connection going. That's why explaining the symptoms of the disease is so important, so the child doesn't think that he or she is the problem.

### Respect How Your Child Processes Information

Since all children process information differently, use your child's individual personality and temperament to inform how you talk to them about your loved one. Megan categorizes children into two main groups: information seekers and information avoiders. The information seekers feel calmer and more secure when they have all the details, which is why they ask a lot of questions, look for explanations, and want to see things firsthand.

"You can identify these kids at a young age, even before a loved one gets sick, because they've always wanted a lot of information," Megan explains. "For them, knowledge is a way of controlling uncertainty." For example, if you're going on a family vacation, they want to know what time you'll arrive and what the destination is going to look like. When they go to the doctor for their annual well visit, they'll ask exactly what's going to happen during the appointment and might watch closely when they get a shot, wanting to understand every step. When a loved one is ill, these children need detailed explanations. They may want to understand the treatment plan and know how things are expected to progress.

"When information seekers feel involved and informed, it helps reduce their anxiety," says Megan. "It's important to be patient with them and provide honest answers, using language they can understand. For these children, leaving out details can create more stress."

In contrast, information avoiders want the bare minimum, since too many details can heighten their anxiety. These children may shy away from conversations about difficult topics and are less likely to ask questions. For example, when going on vacation, an information avoider probably won't ask how or what time you'll get there. At the doctor's office, they might not want to know what's going to happen and will likely look away when they get a shot, avoiding the process altogether. When dealing with a loved one's illness, information avoiders benefit from a more scaled-back approach. Rather than overwhelming them with too much information, share just the key points—what's happening and if things are going to be okay.

"Respecting their need for fewer details helps ease their anxiety while ensuring they still feel supported and included in the conversation," says Megan.

Be clear and straightforward. "You may have noticed that Dad needs more rest. That's because his medicine makes him tired." Then ask if they want to talk more about what you've shared and end by telling them that they can come to you if they have any questions. Information avoiders might not ask questions right away, but it's important to let them know they can talk to you anytime and that no topic is off-limits.

"By giving them space to process in their own way, you can reduce their stress and help them feel secure," says Megan.

As you can see from this book, I'm an information seeker and sharer, so I was surprised to learn that both of my girls only want small doses of information. I respect their process and continually remind them that there's nothing they can't ask me and that there isn't any topic that is off-limits.

Again, regardless of which group your child falls into, seeker or avoider, always update your child if anything changes, such as if surgery is needed or your loved one will undergo new treatment.

## *Finish with Four Key Pieces of Information*

No matter your child's age, personality, or temperament, there are four key things to include when sharing the news of a diagnosis:

- **"You cannot catch this disease. It's not contagious."** Kids associate sickness with a cold or the flu, which they know are contagious. If you don't spell this out, even to adolescents or teens, they may get sick and think, *Do I have what Mommy has?*

- **"You didn't cause it. There's nothing that you did or didn't do that made Dad sick."** Because children of all ages are egocentric, they think, *Did I make Dad sick when I talked back the other day?* Or *Did Mommy get sick because I didn't clean my room?*

- **"You can't control it. There's nothing you can do to change this diagnosis."** Some kids may think, *If I'm a good girl every single day and do exactly what I'm supposed to, that will make Mommy better.*

- **"You will always be safe and taken care of."** When one parent is sick or going to die, a child worries about who is going to take care of them if the well parent gets sick. "Easing that worry at the onset is very important," Megan says. Young kids may even ask, "What if something happens to *you*?" Calmly explain that you're not worried about that and you're there and will keep them safe. Then add that if something *were* to happen, someone else would be there to take care of them. For example, "You have Grandma or Aunt Liz." The goal is to make sure your kids know that they will always be taken care of.

My kids worried about me getting sick. Having grown up with a single mom and not much close family, I totally understood where they were coming from. I was always so scared that something would happen to my mom. So I reassured my girls by saying that I am taking care of myself (this actually is a big motivator for me) and that this was not something I was concerned about.

## HOW TO SUPPORT YOUR CHILD

There's that expression that "actions speak louder than words." This applies to many things in life, including parenting while caregiving. It's not just what you say about your person's illness that impacts your children; your actions matter, too. Here are some expert insights on ways to support your child through this difficult time.

### *Bring Joy to the Journey*

It's important to remind your children that there is still love and joy and happiness to be found.

"Whenever we introduce a stressor to a child, we should find ways to end on a positive note because that will leave their brains in a better space," explains Megan.

You can do this by saying, "We can still live a happy life as a family. We can still do things with Dad that bring us joy." Then you can list things that they love to do with that parent. For example, "We can still cuddle on the couch or watch college football together." Or ask your child what he or she loves to do with the other parent. Then make sure to include those things as often as possible.

"This teaches them that, yes, things are different, and this is sad, but there's still joy to be had," says Megan.

For example, Bruce used to love going to the farmer's market for seasonal fruits and veggies, and he always enjoyed supporting our local farmers. While it's harder to bring him into crowded areas now, that doesn't stop the girls and me from going. When we're there, we make sure to pick up some of his favorite items and bring them home so the girls can enjoy sharing their bounty with him. It's different, but it's still meaningful for us in a new way.

"Children need to have fun in order to grow their nervous systems, and they also need to feel cherished and experience good feelings, not be somber in the house constantly," adds my therapist, Kathleen.

"An important message I like children and parents to have: It takes *practice* to be present with moments of joy *especially* during difficult times, such as illness in the family. Mindfulness techniques, focusing on small moments of happiness, and learning to acknowledge uncomfortable thoughts and emotions without letting them be all-consuming are ways to begin this practice of experiencing moments of joy," says Danielle.

### Give Feelings the Green Light

"Big uncomfortable emotions triggered by a loved one's illness can often get the best of us and that's okay, too! Helping children to have self-compassion and accept their big feelings can help them be better able to experience joy," says Danielle. No matter how old they are, it's important to give your child room to experience the spectrum of emotions they're encountering, and to make sure they don't feel ashamed of what they're feeling.

You can do this by mirroring their emotions. If your child is crying, say, "I see that you are crying and feel really sad. That's okay. I feel sad about this, too."

Along these lines, it's also important for us as parents to share our feelings.

"If your kids see you cry or feel angry, it shows them that it's safe to have these emotions and that they don't have to be strong and brave all the time," Megan explains.

My girls have seen me experience every emotion—the good, the bad, and the extremely ugly, and some I hope they were too young to remember. In those early days of the diagnosis, I was in a state of mourning and therefore very fragile. I didn't shield that from them because it was our reality. Also, they could see and feel my love for their father, my husband, and there was beauty in that. As I settled into what was and worked on processing my feelings in therapy, I was better equipped and able to answer their questions and validate their emotions without breaking down and making this just about myself.

Like many aspects of parenting, it's a balancing act. I want them to know how I feel but also don't want them to think they have to help me get through a rough moment or protect me from their grief and sadness. I'm their mother, not the other way around.

## Have Go-To Responses

Often, well-meaning people ask me about Bruce. I like to have go-to responses prepared so that I don't have to think about it and get emotional or too spun out. I've encouraged my girls to do the same thing so when people ask how their dad is doing, they are not caught off guard or feel like they have to make something up. "Navigating questions from others about a parent's illness can be challenging, and children are entitled to their privacy when deciding what they feel comfortable sharing. Having a prepared response can help them feel more in control and reduce discomfort in social situations," says Danielle.

Help your children develop simple, reassuring answers and practice them in advance. While responses should be age-appropriate and aligned with the child's comfort level, a good approach is to acknowledge the question, provide a brief update if desired, and, if necessary, redirect the conversation. For example: "He's doing okay this week, and resting a lot. Thanks for asking. How was your trip to the beach last weekend?"

## See the Good

As the parent of two school-aged children navigating their dad's young-onset diagnosis, I was encouraged by someone from AFTD to connect with Diana Shulla Cose. Diana is the founding executive director of Lorenzo's House, an organization named after her husband that supports the daughters, sons, and families impacted by young-onset dementia. Her perspective on parenting while caregiving for her husband, Lorenzo, is both profound and deeply relatable.

At the beginning of my carer journey, I wish I'd known someone who shared my family's profile: younger, with young kids (ours were nine and thirteen when Lorenzo was diagnosed), and a partner with dementia. A connection with someone who could share stories, resources, and strategies would have made my journey less isolating and more empowering. While my family and friends showed love, they just couldn't understand and there were few support structures for us. The stigma that dementia is an older person's condition permeated, and I felt left behind.

In the beginning, I felt so sorrowful. I was scared and isolated, and the more Lorenzo changed, the more we lost our way. One night, our older son said, "Mom, you need to stop crying." This was a defining moment for me. I realized that not only were our sons losing their papa, but they were also losing the mom they knew. Unbeknownst to me, I was changing, too. It was time to get organized, own this new identity, and rethink how we could make our family work.

I also realized that our sons' experiences were very different than mine. I didn't know what it felt like to be a son losing a father this way. At times they would look to care for me and my pain—while also caring for their father. Often, they would under-share their wonderings and fears to alleviate more pressure on me.

Inside this upheaval, I was determined to find bits of light and make it a part of our family's DNA. For example,

- We looked for sacred spaces every day—moments where bits of light found us.

- We filled the kitchen cabinet with mugs that read *See the Good*, a mindful mantra.

- We replaced our family dining table with a pool table, a lounge in our own home.

- We placed a marble bistro table near the window. While we wouldn't make it to Paris together in this lifetime, we could go every morning in our own home.

- We made music our medicine, endlessly playing in our home.

- Above all, our greatest tool was love. We showed love—in old, new, and restored ways.

Families walking with younger-onset dementia are unseen, misunderstood, under-resourced; we are undiagnosed and misdiagnosed.

As a result, in 2021, I moved on from a twenty-five-year role in urban education and founded Lorenzo's House, a virtual organization, a sanctuary for families. A place to be seen and understood, a place to belong where we can find each other to both heal in community and advocate for dementia justice. Now I understand the strength and empowerment we feel when connected with others who share our similar journey.

## *Get Ready to Talk About Death*

Death is associated with decline, loss, and the unknown, things that many people are uncomfortable facing. This discomfort translates into silence around end-of-life topics, making them taboo. I used to be part of that silence, purposely avoiding thinking about death and having those conversations. I think this is because I wasn't taught how to navigate grief or talk about death. It's no one's fault, it's just the way things were in my day and age. But Bruce's illness has forced me to confront these subjects, giving me a beautiful opportunity to discuss them more openly with our kids when the opportunity presents itself, which will hopefully break that cycle. Talking about death and grief won't make loss easier, but it does allow room for healing, connection, and a deeper understanding of life's fragility and beauty.

Of course, I didn't always feel this way. My first instinct as a parent is to shield and protect my kids, especially from anything sad or frightening. But as Megan has reminded me:

> We can't shield them from every hard truth. Life includes both joy and loss, and while it's tempting to avoid conversations about difficult topics like death or illness, this can leave children to piece together their own understanding—often leading to fear, confusion, or misconceptions. Children are naturally observant and perceptive, and if we don't guide these conversations, they will find their answers elsewhere, often in ways that leave us out of the narrative.

When a child hears that a parent is sick, he or she will usually ask if that parent is going to die, a common question no matter how old the child is.

"From a really young age, kids have some concept of death, whether they really understand what that means or not," says Megan. "They know that it exists, so we have to explain it in a way that they can understand."

For younger children, you may have to clarify that the person doesn't come back, and we don't see them again. You may tell them that a person's body stops working. Teens and older children are probably more familiar with death and may not need as much explaining.

For kids of all ages, if a disease is terminal but this won't happen for years, you can say, "Yes, your dad will die from this disease, but not right now, so that's not something we're worried about at this moment," or "There are things that Daddy can take that will help him feel better, but there's no cure for what he has and no medicine that can fix his sickness. But this is not something we're worried about right now. If anything changes, I will let you know." That phrase, "if anything changes, I will let you know" is crucial because it eases a child's fear of the unknown, builds trust, lets them know they won't be blindsided by sudden changes, and helps contain anxiety so they can focus on the present rather than worry about what's ahead.

Even more crucial is to follow through with that promise, so if something *does* shift or change, fill them in. This way, nothing is a surprise.

"If you're not truthful and then the parent dies or something happens that you didn't share, you're creating anxiety in the child and a break in trust," Megan says. Then they may think, *I didn't know about this. I was surprised. So what other things are going to happen that I don't know about?*

We create more worries when we're not being honest.

### Read All About It

There are several great children's books that explain diseases in ways children can process. This is especially good if you're not a great communicator, because the books give you language that you might not come up with on your own.

Books can also help your child tell his or her friends or even their whole class if that's something they want to share.

"I had a pediatric patient who had a new diagnosis, and she wanted to tell her first-grade class, but didn't know how," Megan explains. "So we found a book she loved on the subject and she read it to her class to help explain what she was going through. That can be so helpful for kids because it empowers them with words and stories they can share."

A trip to the library or search online can help you find these books for various ages. Also, some organizations offer these resources. For example, the Alzheimer's Association has info to help both young kids and teenagers understand dementia.

### Don't Do It Alone

At this point in the book, you know that you can't caregive alone. You certainly can't parent while caregiving alone either.

"Identify safe people for your kids, like an aunt, a close friend, a cousin," Megan says. Ask your children, "Who else do you feel safe talking to about this?" or "If you feel like you can't come to me, who would you want to go to?" Then reach out to those people and tell them they are on your kids' safe list. If there are certain topics that you don't want these people to discuss with your kids, be clear about that. Most people will be flattered and happy to help, and bringing in this community creates more safety nets for your children. My kids have the right support in place, and we've identified people in their lives they can talk to about anything they don't want to bring my way. This makes me feel good knowing that others have their backs, too.

No matter what grade they are in, your child's school is another important community.

"Kids are at school for six to seven hours a day, so you want feet on the ground who can watch them and reach out to you if there are any behavioral changes," says Megan. "It's also another place for them to go if they're feeling sad. For example, they can meet with a school counselor, which expands your toolbox of people who can help support your children as they navigate their grief and sadness so it's not just falling on you."

If you have a very sensitive kid who needs added support, a therapist, as we learned, can help. Megan suggests a play therapist for younger kids and talk therapy for adolescents and teens. There are also a ton of great resources and programs such as groups, associations, and camps for kids.

Identifying your kids' community can also help you find people to lean on when you're feeling overwhelmed. They can assist with things like homework, school, and activity drop-offs, buying snacks for a class party, or helping older kids with driving lessons or college applications. They can also watch your person so you can be with your kids.

"The biggest mistake I see parents make is not asking for help and not asking for it soon enough. Caregivers, especially those who are parents, feel like asking for help means they're relinquishing some control and that can feel scary when you're dealing with sickness and diseases that are changing," says Megan. "Yet, when we don't seek help, we risk losing even more control and unintentionally adding to the chaos."

## *Say Goodbye to Guilt*

Although I've talked about guilt in Chapter 6, it definitely deserves a mention in a chapter about parenting while caregiving. Having a family was always my greatest dream. Growing up, I had such a clear vision of the kind of mother I wanted to be: calm, collected, and patient. (All the things that don't come that easy to me!) I imagined creating the ideal environment for my children. When my daughters came along, I felt incredibly blessed that I had the resources to offer them everything I didn't have growing up in a single-parent household, like music lessons, their choice of activities, and participation in sports teams with travel opportunities. I envisioned myself being fully engaged, taking them to every event, Bruce and me cheering from the sidelines, dividing and conquering, and making sure they had everything they needed to succeed.

What I never anticipated was that I would find myself in the middle of caregiving, juggling not only the needs of my children but those of someone else, and that my perfect dream would have to change. As those opportunities for the girls' activities arose, reality set in. The weight of caregiving, on top of parenting, began to overwhelm me. What I thought I could manage quickly became too much to handle. I found myself unable to follow through with all those commitments as there just wasn't enough of me to go around. With that came the guilt. Guilt that I wasn't the parent I envisioned and that I couldn't just "buck up" and do it all. I felt like I was letting my children down, not giving them the opportunities I had dreamed for them. I wanted to be everything for everyone, but in trying to do so, I lost sight of what was truly sustainable for me as a parent.

If you can relate to this, remind yourself that your kids had no clue how high you set that bar for yourself. Mine certainly didn't. Also, know that you are trying your best, but as Evelyn would say, "life started life-ing." As I learned from Dr. Sadeghi, I trust that all of this is happening for us and not to us. I'm doing the best that I can. And so are you.

## Caring for You = Caring for Your Kids

As we've learned again and again, it's essential to care for yourself during this time, not only for you but for your kids as well. When you don't, it becomes harder to look after them, and they notice when you're exhausted, down, and low energy. Think again about the message given by flight attendants to put your oxygen mask on first before helping anyone.

"As parents and caregivers, we often lose ourselves in the effort to keep everything together," says Megan. "But the truth is, you can't hold everything together unless you're taking care of yourself. We need to shift the narrative—caring for yourself isn't neglecting others; it's what allows you to care for them even better."

Everyone copes differently, so figure out what calms and renews you; is it watching a movie alone, reading, or meditating? It doesn't have to be extreme, but it does have to be something that fills you up again. (See Chapter 4 for more suggestions.)

This is also crucial for helping your kids cope with life's ups and downs because you're modeling how to prioritize your well-being. You're telling them, "I'm taking care of me so I can take really good care of you. I'm taking care of me so that I have energy to do all the fun things that we love to do together." You can even spell it out for them. Say, "I feel really sad right now so I'm going to take ten minutes and be by myself to take some deep breaths, and then I'm going to come back out and feel better." The goal of you modeling this is for them to grow up thinking, "I'm feeling this way today. I'm going to go take a moment to myself and do something that makes me feel better." Showing your child that you can process your emotions by making time for yourself and come back feeling renewed is priceless and life-changing for them.

### Model Not Coping, Too

We are never going to be perfect, especially in high-stress situations, so we also need to model that it's okay to get upset or mad because we all hit our limits and have bad days. Give yourself grace. These are difficult times. There is a lot going on. It is okay to lose your cool. It is okay to mess up and to make mistakes. It's what you do afterward that matters.

When you have those moments, "apologize, acknowledge what you did, and validate the feelings you hurt," Megan explains. It's as simple as saying, "I got really mad and said some things that I probably shouldn't have said. I'm sorry. I'm going to mess up. This isn't going to be the last time, but I'm going to try really hard next time because I know that it makes you sad, and that makes me sad." Another option is to say, "I'm feeling really overwhelmed and sad about Dad today, and that's making me grumpy. I'm sorry." The good news is that this is a teachable moment because it shows your kids that even when they mess up, they're still going to be loved and taken care of.

There are times when I can feel myself boiling over and I snap at the kids. I feel so awful afterward, but I have learned the art of accountability and apology. I say what happened and why, and "I'm sorry" with no ifs, ands, or buts attached. It's been incredible to see the girls do the same when they have a snappy moment with me or each other. Although I feel like I mess up as a parent all the time, these moments remind me that at least I'm doing something right.

I also let the girls know that I've never been a parent before and the scenarios and situations I'm navigating as a parent and caregiver are all new. I feel like I'm making it all up as I go! That allows them to understand that I am human and I'm not on some parental pedestal, so I don't have that far to fall.

### Give Kids Some Control

Kids want control. They strive for it. So find little areas where they can have a say within boundaries. One area is asking your children which friends they would like to tell about their sick loved one.

"Give them some autonomy over who gets to know and, if they want, allow them to tell those friends themselves. You can be there to support or just role-play with them where you're his or her friend and she's telling them about the situation," Megan says.

Also, if your kids don't want to tell their friends, make it clear that that's okay, too. Just say, "If you don't want to talk about it with your friends right now, that's okay. Let me know when you're ready to share." You can also give your kids control over . . .

- **How much they want to know about what's going on:**
  Ask, *Would you like to know more about Dad's treatment,*

*or do you want me to share updates only if something big happens?*

- **How they want to spend time with your person:** Ask, *Do you want to watch a show with Mom or just sit and talk?*

- **Which small caregiving tasks they can help with:** Suggest they might like picking which blanket Mom will have today or what snack to make Dad.

- **How they will express themselves:** Suggest they might talk to you or a professional therapist, write in a journal, or draw.

## *Include Your Loved One*

As Evelyn has watched Bruce's disease progress, she's shared how she wishes she'd appreciated their time together more when things were different. She often says that if she'd known how much their relationship would change, she wouldn't have taken those moments for granted. What I've tried to help her understand is that we can't know what we don't know, and that's okay. Just because we didn't realize how precious those moments were at the time doesn't mean they weren't meaningful. Bruce enjoyed those times, and they remain good memories for all of us.

One way to keep memories alive is to look at old photos, share stories, and create something out of those memories.

The girls and I love scrolling through my phone to see photos and videos of them when they were younger. It's a beautiful reminder of our time with Bruce.

Take time to reminisce about your loved one with your kids and invite friends and family to do the same. Mabel loves to hear stories about her dad, and I'll tell you, there is nothing better than a Bruce Willis story. I love telling them and sitting there after, just laughing. Bruce really was a total trip, pure fun and love.

"Take meaningful photos from a time when your loved one was still very much themselves and create something—whether it's a painting, a montage, or a video," Megan suggests. For example, create photo albums so those memories don't just stay tucked away in a digital cloud.

Keeping our loved one's spirit and essence alive in ways that feel meaningful and appropriate allows us and our kids to hold on to the joy the loved one brought into our lives. It helps ensure we remember who they were before the illness, not just who they've become because of it. Finding this balance lets us honor our person's full story while making room for both love and grief.

Here are some other ideas and projects you can do with your kids:

- **Memory Boxes:** Create a memory box filled with meaningful items connected to their loved one, like favorite keepsakes, small objects, or handwritten notes that reflect their personality, hobbies, and important life events. This can be a tactile way for kids and family to connect with their loved one's legacy.

- **Personalized Playlists:** Create a playlist of your loved one's favorite songs or music from their era. Music has a unique way of connecting us emotionally, and this can be comforting for both the loved one and their caregivers.

- **Story Journals:** Encourage kids and other family members to write down memories, anecdotes, or endearing things your loved one has said or done. This journal can be a keepsake for generations. You can also send an email to friends, family, and even business associates of your loved one to collect their stories, too. It's a beautiful way to celebrate your person's life beyond the illness and create a fuller picture of him or her and the impact he or she had.

## The Caveat to "Kids Are So Resilient"

We often hear that kids are so resilient, and this is a fact I've found comfort in. However, Megan explains that "while kids are resilient, resiliency is also taught." In other words, kids learn resiliency from their parents, so it's important to model how to care for someone who is sick while caring for yourself, and how to caregive but still show up and have fun.

"This teaches our children that we cannot avoid bad things, but we can choose how we react to those bad things," Megan says. "In other words, we don't get a choice on *if* suffering exists or not, but we *do* get a say in how we react to that suffering. That is a gift that we can give our children, the gift of resiliency and teaching them how to overcome challenging and scary situations."

CAREGIVING WHILE PARENTING is hard. It's not something you'd wish for. But you're here, and I hope you can take comfort in the fact that you're teaching your kids life lessons that are going to serve them well in the future, helping them build resilience, empathy, and the strength to navigate life's inevitable obstacles. And I hope you can all find some joy along the way.

## QUESTIONS AND ANSWERS
## WITH MEGAN GRAHAM

As I've mentioned, Megan was truly instrumental in helping me navigate the difficult path of caregiving while parenting. Her insight made me feel less alone and has allowed me to communicate more effectively with my girls.

**What are some practical tips parents can immediately apply to help their children navigate a loved one's illness?**

- **Maintain routine.** Predictability provides security, even in uncertain times.

- **Check in regularly.** Even brief conversations can open the door for deeper discussions. For kids who can read and write, a box that is at the center of the home where they can write and leave messages at any time, and where you can leave answers, can be helpful for those who are having a hard time verbally expressing themselves.

- **Take care of yourself.** It's crucial to prioritize your own well-being so you can remain emotionally present for your child. Set aside time to take care of yourself—even short breaks can recharge your energy—and lean on other people. Talking to others who understand your experience can provide valuable emotional relief and practical advice.

**How can you use play to communicate and connect with your children during this time?**

Children often express their emotions through play. Joining in their play not only strengthens your bond but also gives you insight into how they're processing the situation. For example, if they're playing with dolls or action figures, they might act out scenarios related to the changes they're observing. You can gently guide or support their play by introducing comforting narratives, like a character helping another who is "forgetful." Engage in creative activities like drawing, storytelling, or role-playing, which provide safe spaces for children to express feelings they may not yet have the words for. Playtime can also be a respite from heavy emotions, offering both you and your child moments of joy and connection.

**What is some language that parents can use to support their kids during this journey?**

Use metaphors or stories to explain complex ideas (e.g., "The medicine is like a superhero fighting the bad cells in Dad's body"). Here are some examples based on developmental age for children who have a parent with FTD or Alzheimer's disease:

- **For young children (ages 4–7):** "Sometimes you might see Mommy get upset or confused. That's because her brain is having trouble figuring things out. It's not your fault."

- **For middle childhood (ages 8–12):** "Sometimes you might notice Mom gets upset or repeats herself. It's okay to feel frustrated or sad about that. It's a hard thing to go through, and I'm here to talk if you need me."

- **For teens (ages 13+):** "Mom has a condition called fronto-temporal dementia. It's a disease that affects her brain and changes how she thinks, feels, and acts. It's not her fault, and it's not something she can control."

## *Something to think about . . .*

What's one insight from this chapter that you can use to help your children?

_____

_____

_____

_____

_____

_____

_____

_____

_____

_____

_____

_____

_____

_____

# EIGHT

# Bringing In Help

It's the smart person who gets help, not the weak one.

**DANIEL AMEN,**
*MD, founder of the Amen Clinics*

While writing this book, when I asked experts for their top piece of advice for care partners, no matter their field of expertise, they said to get help. And when I asked about the biggest mistake care partners make on this journey, they said it's not getting that help soon enough.

This is something I wish I knew earlier. Actually, I wish I'd known that I was allowed to ask for support and that I was not a failure because I needed it. The idea that we must always be strong and self-sufficient has been ingrained in us by society, especially for women. In the process, we've lost our sense of true community and shared support. Asking for help can feel like we've failed as caregivers or we're admitting weakness, when it's really a sign of wisdom and strength.

The hard truth is this: We can't caregive alone, and it shouldn't be presumed that we have to. Most of us come into this new role with no medical expertise, we're just learning on the fly. And at some point, your loved one's medical needs may surpass what you feel equipped or confident enough to handle, or your home may not be set up in a way that fully supports you in meeting those needs. In those situations, getting help is essential, whether that looks like family and friends stepping in, formal caregiving, a day program in your area, memory-care assisted living, or a skilled nursing facility, among other options. You must bring people into the fold to support you.

Now, you may be shaking your head or thinking, *I'm my person's partner/child/spouse/fill-in-the-blank. I'm supposed to do it all*, or *No one can do it like I would*, or *My person won't adapt to someone else. I need to protect my person's dignity.* I know this because I had every single one of those thoughts and fought against having help for a long time, a *really* long time.

"Caregivers spend so many months or years managing daily medications, therapies, and interventions, and understand these routines down to the finest detail. They know their loved one's preferences and moods and how to intervene if they're having a bad day or unexpected difficulty," says Dr. Sadeghi. "Because they've become experts in this care, they don't believe anyone else can provide it at the same level."

That was me. I had it all down to a fine science and felt it was my duty as Bruce's wife to do everything. I was convinced that no one knew him or could care for him better. Plus, I take great pride in being his care partner. To me, this isn't just about meeting his physical needs, it's about showing up for him in a way that reflects the love and commitment we've built over the years. It's about honoring the life we've shared, the man he's been, and the family we've created together. There's something deeply meaningful about being the person he relies on, even as it challenges me in ways I never expected. It's a privilege to witness his moments of clarity, his quiet strength, and the unique ways he still expresses his love for us. Caring for him has taught me patience, resilience, and the true depth of unconditional love. And through it all, he's faced this disease with the strength and grit of the badass he's always been.

Yet, in all of that, I wouldn't be human if I didn't say it's frightfully difficult and traumatic and that I needed help. Not only was I juggling all the caregiving duties, but I was the primary parent to our kids. I was also diligently trying to protect our privacy, so it was hard for me to trust and let someone in. But what I didn't realize was that someone else *can* learn, and people can be trusted. They can get to know your person, and your person can adapt to them. It just requires a little patience, time, trial, and error.

Eventually, I did raise my hand and ask for help. It was a hard decision and something I was very self-conscious about in the beginning, but I'm at peace with it now because I see how beneficial it was for our family. Asking for help saved us in more ways than one. I'm deeply grateful to someone close to this situation, someone I trusted, who gave me the "permission" to ask for help, permission I didn't even realize I needed. They reassured me that it was okay, that I wasn't a bad person or failing by admitting that I would soon be out of my depth.

I'm sharing this part of my story with you, in all its vulnerability, in case it helps you feel less alone and gives you the courage to seek the help you need and deserve. And if you're like me and feel like you need someone to give you permission to get help, then let me be that person for you.

## CREATE A MEDICAL FOLDER

It's important that you are not the *only* person who is up-to-date on your loved one's medical info. I remember filling up Bruce's pill organizer and thinking it was a little scary that I was the only one who knew his medicine routine. In fact, I was the only one who knew most of his medical information, such as doctors, appointments, insurance, etc. At the time I didn't realize that I should share this with others in case something happened to me. The hard truth here is that life can throw unexpected curveballs. It's serious, scary, and un-pleasant to think about, but it's a reality. So please make sure to write down your person's medical information and give it to someone else—a family member, a friend, another care-giver. I suggest creating a folder—either digital or hard copy—where you compile all information related to your person's condition, including his or her schedule, names and doses of medications, pharmacy, insurance, doctors' names and numbers, and reports from previous tests or appoint-ments, and then make sure someone else has access to it.

## ASSEMBLING YOUR CARE TEAM

"Emma, you don't have someone in your home at night?" Bruce's neurologist asked me at one appointment.

"No," I said. It was something I'd never even thought about.

"Well, you know what? It's time," she told me. "You have stairs in your house and other things that can affect Bruce's safety and that of your family. Plus, *you* need to get some sleep. It's not healthy."

"No," I said, shaking my head. "Having someone around at night is very complicated for us."

"You will get used to it," she urged. "Remember, this is a progressive disease and the sooner you bring someone in, the better it will be for everyone."

I sighed.

"You're one of the lucky ones because you have the resources to hire someone," she added. "You can't do this alone, and you don't need to."

This was not the first time I'd heard that I needed to get help caregiving, although no one had mentioned nighttime help. All the doctors I'd talked to had said some version of this to me because they knew the weight and complications that FTD brings and what I was experiencing, how much I was taking on while raising our young daughters, and what was to come. Yet, no matter how many times I heard it, I refused. That was, until our neurologist explained that we were approaching a level that wasn't safe for Bruce, our young children, or me. It was the true wake-up call I needed.

## Introducing the Support Person

When you first bring in a support person, introduce them to your loved one as a helper, someone who will handle a few tasks, like driving or lending an extra set of hands. This approach can make the transition feel smoother for everyone involved. For me, in our privilege, I called our new caregiver an "assistant," and Bruce, ever mindful of ensuring I was supported, agreed without hesitation. In fact, he even seemed to welcome the extra layer of help, which made things easier to navigate at first.

If you feel your loved one might be apprehensive or you know there could be some pushback, here are some other ways you can frame it. And remember, this is for *you* to be able to get some relief so you can continue being the best care partner possible. You can tell your loved one that the new person is a:

- **Household helper:** "This is someone who will help out around the house with things I can't always get to." Or "They're here to make life a little easier for both of us."

- **Friend or companion:** "This is someone who can keep you company when I'm busy or running errands." Or "I thought it might be nice to have someone around to chat with or watch a show together."

- **Support for you:** "This is someone who's helping me stay on top of everything at home so I can focus more on us." Or "They're helping me manage the day-to-day so we can spend more quality time together."

Some people worry about saying these things because they feel like they're lying. But as dementia care specialist Teepa Snow explains, "There's a difference between telling the truth, the whole truth, and nothing but the truth—which could be something that the person can neither accept nor understand—and telling the truth that is within the bounds of accuracy."

A white lie would be saying, "The person coming in is just going to visit today, and then you'll never have to see them again." But the truth is that you *are* hiring the person for the above reasons—household helper, support for you, or as a companion because you can't do it all alone anymore.

"That is accurate. But to say out loud to your loved one, 'The reason I'm hiring this person is because you're not competent anymore' would be cruel and not helpful to either one of you," adds Teepa.

## *Letting Go of Perfection*

Now, I understand that getting help might feel like a big adjustment. Here's the challenge: Sometimes FTD or other forms of dementia can bring moments of agitation or frustration. Seeing your loved one distressed can be so upsetting that your immediate instinct is to jump in and smooth things over.

But doing so too quickly doesn't allow the formal caregiver, friend, or family member the opportunity to learn how to connect with your loved one and find their own rhythm. I learned this the hard way. Each time I stepped in on anything, because I was programmed to, I unintentionally reset the process, leaving us all feeling frustrated. I do give myself some grace here because we had young children at home and I wanted to do my best to keep things as level and steady as possible for them. It's truly a dance, and at first, it may feel like everyone's stepping on each other's toes.

Looking back, I realized that, like I said before, patience and a little grit are essential. By allowing yourself to ride out the learning curve, taking some deep breaths, and letting go of perfectionism, you'll see that the support person you've brought in for your loved one will eventually find his or her rhythm, and when they do, it brings tremendous relief.

## REDEFINING HOME

As Bruce's disease progressed, doctors and specialists gave me a sense of what the future would look like. It was clear to me as well. I wanted to preserve so much for Bruce and the girls, but the smoke and mirrors I was creating for them would only grow harder to maintain as time went on. Although we can't protect our kids from everything in life, there are certain things we should shield them from if it's in our control, and this was something that was in my control for once. I kept going back to the idea of *What would Bruce want me to do? How would he want me to handle this situation? What would I want Bruce to do if this was ME?* Knowing your loved one's values and belief system makes difficult calls like this easier to navigate even when the decisions we need to make are unimaginable and hard to fathom.

The truth was that Mabel and Evelyn's daily lives were being turned upside down. For example, with FTD and other forms of dementia, some people become more sensitive to noise, which can cause distraction, confusion, and agitation. So I had everyone tiptoeing around the house to keep it as peaceful and serene as possible. This meant playdates were obsolete and forget about sleepovers. It was like I had a muzzle on our children, and I felt like I was starting to isolate them from having their own lives. But when I thought about how loud and crazy and fun Bruce loved to be with his girls, his music blaring, I realized I was creating an environment he never would have wanted, and this made me feel awful for all of us. I know his values, what's important to him, and that his five daughters always came first. Anyone who knows Bruce knows that his love for his girls was unwavering, and he cared deeply about their happiness and well-being. In fact, you don't even have to know Bruce to understand that he is truly a family man. He wanted the best for Mabel and Evelyn and a home where they could be kids. At the time, that was not the case, and it wasn't benefiting anyone. Our home became a place where no one was thriving. I knew I needed to find a better balance and fit for all of us, honoring what Bruce would have wanted while protecting the girls from the unnecessary added stress.

I decided it was in our family's best interest to find a second home near ours where Bruce could live with the right support and comfort he needed.

Bruce living in our second family home was not an easy decision. In fact, it was the hardest one I've had to make so far on this journey, and it was difficult to tell our kids. But I'd been honest with them every step of the way, and this moment was no exception.

"We've come to a point in Daddy's disease where the care he requires is changing. It has to be more tailored to his every need," I told them. "And you should be in a home that is more tailored to *your* needs now."

"Also, Daddy would want you to have playdates, sleepovers, and more freedom than you've been able to have here. That would make him so happy," I added.

I assured them that where Bruce would be living would be our second home, too, a place they'd keep personal things like toys, arts and crafts supplies, bathing suits, pj's, and games, and that we could go stay with him anytime they wanted. Even though they'd lived with his disease for so long that they understood, and even though this decision ensures Bruce's overall well-being and safety and allows our young children to thrive, it was an uncertain and painful time for us. In fact, it's still painful for me. After all, this is my husband, and having him in another home was not part of the future we'd mapped out together. You really can't dream this stuff up.

I've wrestled with whether or not to share this part of my journey. Guilt and shame have weighed heavily on me, and I've had to work through these emotions. But I've come to believe that sharing this serves a greater purpose: to remind caregivers that love isn't measured by where care happens but by the care itself. Every family's needs are different, and there is no single "right way" to do this. If any part of our story can help another person navigate their own, then it's worth sharing. The lessons I've learned in this experience feel important to pass along, and I hope that by opening up, it resonates with you or offers you reassurance about your own choices.

Will I be judged? Most likely. Especially by those who have opinions but no real experience with FTD, let alone while raising young children around it. Unfortunately, judgment seems to come with the caregiving territory, which is exactly why I feel compelled to share. I'm going to throw myself in front of that bullet. It's time to shift these narratives and judgments, whether they come from those who haven't walked in our shoes or even from those who have. And if our family's story is going to be shared, I'd rather it come from me, in a way that is true and authentic, rather than risk a harmful and inaccurate narrative being shaped by others.

It has not been easy, and the truth is I would love to return to my old life with my husband and kids pre-FTD. But that's not in the cards for us and we have habituated to it over time. Now I rest easy knowing without a doubt that this is what Bruce would want. Regardless, I remain Bruce's primary caregiver; our second home is warm and safe and allows me to continue giving him the best care possible, while our primary home allows me to give our young girls the focus and attention they deserve.

Yes, I absolutely recognize what a privilege this is. It's as "extra" as it could and should be. While this isn't how I envisioned Bruce's retirement or our life, it has allowed me to give him the very best care, care he worked hard to afford. I feel good knowing that I've been able to put this support system in place for him. In my head, I can hear him saying, "Don't skimp, Emma!" Thankfully, I've been able to see the positive impact this new environment has had on him and the good it has brought to all of us as a family.

When I decided to share this, I thought about an op-ed in *The New York Times* that my friend Patti Davis wrote about Sandra Day O'Connor, the first woman on the Supreme Court, when O'Connor passed away in 2023. Her husband, John, had Alzheimer's disease, and the article talked about how brave and selfless O'Connor had been to openly share her decision to put John in a memory care facility. This was the early 2000s, when not many people were discussing Alzheimer's or dementia, and if they were, it was in hushed tones. Also, the idea of publicly acknowledging the need to place a loved one in care was almost unheard of. I can only imagine the public reaction.

Patti's take on that decision was profound to me, and I took it to heart. She wrote, "I so admired Sandra Day O'Connor's openness, and I imagined the thousands of people in similar situations who felt gratitude that someone was shining a light on a dilemma that so many suffer through in the shadows."

When I read that, I thought about how there is still so much judgment and stigma today that surrounds the decision to place your loved one in an assisted-living memory care or skilled nursing facility that provides safe and appropriate care for them and you. However, sometimes what is required for your person goes beyond your capabilities as a care partner. And yet that doesn't mean you love them any less. In fact, I don't know if there is anything more loving than making sure that your person has the right attention and that his or her needs are met fully 100 percent of the time. For example, while Bruce might not be in a memory care facility, we've been able to provide a warm and caring environment completely tailored to his needs. And there has been no better feeling than that.

Giving and allowing the girls some space from Bruce also helps prepare them for his death. I know how dark and jarring that sounds, but that is the harsh reality of the world I must navigate to continue to protect our girls the best way I can. (And no, I don't have a specific timeline on this. But what I have learned is that people with FTD have an average life expectancy of seven to thirteen years after the start of symptoms.) This disease of FTD is horrendous, but it gives you a little grace to be able to plan and organize your affairs. I think getting used to it being just the three of us in our home will lessen the shock for Mabel and Evelyn when the inevitable comes. Until there is a cure, this disease will always win.

## How Do You Know It's Time to Get Help, and What Kind of Help?

Arlene Schollaert is family services director at Amazing Place in Houston, a nonprofit organization with a mission to empower families facing the challenges of dementia and Alzheimer's and to advance brain health for all. She states that it can be difficult to know when to hire in-home care or to move your person to an assisted-living or memory care community. The care partner should make this decision when their ability to care for their person alone is no longer sustainable.

That said, this isn't always easy to recognize. When your loved one starts exhibiting more serious symptoms, you might feel so overwhelmed that it's difficult to see the full picture. The stress and worry can wear you down, spilling into everything you do, from caregiving and parenting to simply existing. You might notice yourself becoming easily frustrated with your person and short-fused with your kids, family, and friends. You may feel exhausted, moody, and wound tight or notice that your own health is declining, and it can be hard to imagine how to move forward. This is what Teepa means when she says that without support, you will ultimately lose yourself as much as you lose the other person.

"Your playfulness will disappear. Your pleasure in being alive will disappear. Your sense of being purposeful and valuable will disappear. And you'll be miserable," she says. "And that's *not* required to do this job. So you have to let go of what you can't have anymore, which is that independence to caregive on your own. It requires reaching out and finding support. That's a reality. There's no way around it."

If you are uncertain about needing help, Arlene suggests asking yourself the following questions, which will provide a snapshot of how much support your person now requires and your ability to continue to manage all these needs on your own:

- If your person was in the house alone and there was a fire, would they know how to get out on their own?

- What are the tasks you do for your person that they used to do themselves? Make a list because you may not realize how much you're doing until you see it written down.

- Can you get seven or eight hours of sleep a night?

- Have you dropped all or many of your activities because you just don't have time?

- Have you lost your connections with family and friends?

Here are some questions of my own that I also suggest you ask yourself:

- When was the last time you went to a medical or personal appointment for yourself?

- Do you feel physically or emotionally exhausted most days?

- Have you experienced any feelings of resentment or burnout in your caregiving role?

- If something happened to you, do you have someone who could step in and care for your loved one?

- Do you feel overwhelmed managing medications or medical appointments?

- Is your loved one showing signs of needing more supervision than you can provide alone?

- Have you noticed changes in your own health since becoming a caregiver?

- Are family dynamics creating tension around caregiving responsibilities?

Ultimately, you're doing the best you can. As Arlene explains, "The disease has brought you to this point of needing more support. It's not your lack of love or caring. It's the disease progression. It's *because* of the love and care that you are doing this. It's for yourself, it's for your family, and it's for the person with this disease." Remind yourself of that.

---

"You cannot make good choices for anybody when your brain is fried, you're depleted, you're exhausted, and you aren't yourself. You need a break and space."

**TEEPA SNOW,**
*dementia care specialist, consulting associate at
Duke University's School of Nursing,
and founder of Positive Approach to Care*

---

## *Navigating the High Price Tag*

Before I continue talking about getting help, I have to acknowledge the high cost of bringing in home health care and working with memory-care assisted living and skilled nursing facilities. It's disheartening to see how expensive and inaccessible this kind of support is to so many.

"People are often confined to make choices based on their finances and that is a painful place to be in. We are not where we need to be [in this country] for people to get the support they need," says Lauren Miller Rogen, a screenwriter, director, producer, and cofounder with her husband, actor Seth Rogen, of Hilarity for Charity, a national nonprofit on a mission to care for families impacted by Alzheimer's disease, activate the next generation of Alzheimer's advocates, and be a leader in brain-health research and education. "You should be able to make a choice of how you care for your loved one, whether it's in your home or in a home that is professionally run." There's no way around it: The cost of care, especially care outside your home, can be astronomical. It's one of the main reasons people don't get help.

"People are afraid of the huge cost of this kind of care so they avoid planning for it. But this doesn't make it go away, and often there is planning you can do to make it accessible," explains Katie Brandt of the Frontotemporal Disorders Unit at Massachusetts General Hospital, who suggests finding a certified elder law attorney. Share your values and talk with them about financial planning. They are typically experts in estate planning, wills, and trusts and can help you see that there is a path to getting help. Call and ask, "Have you helped other families navigate financial planning and advanced-care planning after a diagnosis of dementia?" You want someone who specializes in this.

If you don't have the resources to hire help, you may have to get creative about pulling together a support system. Talk to family, friends, and those in your community; reach out to volunteer groups that offer companion services, to the social worker or nurse at your neurologist's office, and to organizations like the Alzheimer's Association (which helps with other forms of dementia as well), AFTD, or your local Area Agency on Aging. For loved ones who were in the armed forces, caregivers can sometimes get help through the Veterans Health Administration.

## *You Are Not Failing Your Person*

One of the biggest reasons care partners resist moving our loved ones out of our own homes is guilt. We think this means that we have failed our person or that we are not doing what he or she wanted because we made a promise to one another.

"Sometimes the person you are caring for was previously involved in looking after another relative, like a grandparent or their own parent, and at the time they said to you, 'I never want to be like that. Don't ever put me in a home,'" explains Katie. "But what your loved one was *really* saying was 'Don't abandon me. Don't leave me alone. Don't forget about me.' They want to know that you're going to be there for them." For me, reframing the situation and seeing it from this perspective gave me a deeper sense of compassion and clarity.

Another thing to consider is that your person may have been a young child when they visited a relative in a nursing home, and they may have a negative memory of that visit. I know when I was growing up, we heard horror stories about these types of homes. But a lot has changed with skilled nursing facilities in the past decades. Chances are, when your loved one expressed their wish to remain at home, both of you were in good health and couldn't have anticipated the level of care that might eventually be needed. You likely didn't imagine that one of you would have to manage things like assisting with showers, addressing incontinence, or physically supporting the other. Even if you made that promise at the start of your caregiving journey, you or your loved one couldn't have known just how challenging it would become.

Remember that when or if you feel this sense of guilt, come back to the advice a lot of experts have shared with me: Sometimes this promise is one you can't keep. You are not breaking it because you are not loving and caring; in fact, you are breaking it because you *are*. You are doing one of the hardest jobs in the world, so try to lift yourself up rather than tear yourself down.

Knowing what I do now, I've created a detailed and legally documented care plan to ensure that my children and the other adults in my life understand the type of care I would want if, God forbid, I'm ever unable to make those decisions myself. No one likes to think about or plan for these situations, but it is important and feels like the right and loving thing to do, especially if it can take the burden and difficult decision-making off the shoulders of your loved ones.

## JUDGMENT IS PAR FOR THE CAREGIVING COURSE—ALTHOUGH IT SHOULDN'T BE

Unfortunately, as we've learned, there is a lot of judgment when it comes to being a care partner, from both within and outside the community. Often when a person moves their loved one out of their home, others will say something along the lines of "I would never do that."

If you hear similar remarks, remind yourself that until the person judging you walks in your dementia-caregiving shoes, they can't fully understand the countless tasks you manage or the needs that remain unmet, both yours and those of your loved one. Even if the people offering their opinions *are* also caregivers, the reality is their experiences are unique to their situations, just as yours is to you. Dementia manifests differently in every person and every home. Every care plan is different, and each person's journey is their own.

"Usually, when people make judgmental comments, it's not about you; it's about them and their own emotions or experiences," Katie explains. She suggests that you invite the judger to come and visit your person while they're engaging with that new service or support so the judgmental person can see its benefits. You can also work with your own mental health provider to decide how much engagement you need and want to have with people who judge your choices. You can't change people's minds, but you can build that strength within yourself to let their comments roll off you and have a thicker skin.

I know it's hard. I've been working on that, too. One thing that has helped me is something called the Let Them Theory, which I learned from Mel Robbins, world-renowned expert on mindset, motivation, and behavior change, host of *The Mel Robbins Podcast*, and author of *The Let Them Theory*.

"The Let Them Theory is about freedom. Two simple words—*Let Them*—will free you from the burden of trying to manage and please other people," Robbins explains. "No matter what happens around you, you decide how it will affect you. You decide if a comment from a loved one destroys your self-esteem or rolls off your back. It's that simple. You have the power." It's a work in progress, but "Let them" is one of the silent mantras I repeat to myself when I feel like I'm being judged.

On that note, I believe society can do better by not judging others when their care plans don't align with your own. We need to shift our mindset to lift care partners up instead of tearing each other down and viewing caregiving as some kind of competition. This is one reason I feel so strongly about sharing this personal part of our journey. My intention is to shine a light on all the different aspects of caregiving that people often feel they need to keep in the dark. I hope that by doing so, other care partners won't have to experience shame, guilt, or even more isolation over decisions that are so personal to their families. And if someone has a hard time with that, then put this book in their hands.

## WHY BRINGING IN HELP HELPS EVERYONE

The decision to bring in support is a hard but essential one on this journey. We cannot do this alone. Otherwise, we will simply burn out, and our loved ones might not receive the care they need as their diseases progress. But there are a few other benefits to bringing in help, some of which might surprise you.

### *You Can Get Back to Being You*

One benefit to getting help, whether you bring it into your home or have your person move to a community-based setting, is the ability to get back to your original role in your person's life.

"There are so many things you can outsource—laundry, medication management, driving or preparing meals; what you *cannot* outsource is being your loved one's spouse, child, sibling, partner, or friend. That's your unique gift and presence in their life," explains Katie. "No one else can sit with your loved one, hold their hand, listen to your wedding song together, and look through family photos. Having someone else do other parts of caregiving increases your emotional bandwidth to show up for your person in your unique role."

"Plug other people in for the easier tasks and save yourself for the critical places and special moments where no one will be as good as you," adds Teepa.

This is something I didn't always understand. Early on in this process, before I started looking for formal caregivers, Sara M., who is on Bruce's medical team, said to me, "Emma, we want to get you back to being Bruce's wife." *His wife?* I thought. *I* am *his wife.* Everything was so blurry to me during that time, I couldn't even wrap my head around what she was saying. That was, until I started to bring in help and support.

Before, I was so stressed out and busy that I could never sit with Bruce and just be. Instead, I was constantly getting up and down, thinking about all the things I needed to do, and on edge. He could feel my stress. As I've mentioned, Dr. Sadeghi has explained to me that those around you are connected to and affected by your Wi-Fi, i.e., the energy you project, even when you're not interacting directly with them. My Wi-Fi wasn't just spotty—it was buffering on a bad connection! Once I brought in help, the signal finally started to strengthen.

Now I get what Sara meant. I can just be Bruce's wife again, and there has been no greater gift.

The other day, Bruce and I sat on the patio of our second home, watching the girls swim and giggle in the pool. As we held hands, Bruce hummed along to the Frank Sinatra song that was playing in the background. For a moment, it was a teeny tiny bit of normalcy that we really needed.

It took me some time to see it that way and reframe it rather than sitting in guilt. But now I can truly enjoy our fleeting time together, and there's nothing I could ever do to repay our care team for that. I'm forever grateful that I get to enjoy Bruce again as his wife and that our kids have their mom back.

### It Brings Your Inner Circle Closer

As I assume you know well by now, I'm an over-functioner and not good at delegating. However, because I was taking on everything, it probably never gave anyone else a chance to help. What I've learned from my therapist, Kathleen, is that when you over-function, it gives everyone else around you the permission to under-function. You are sending a loud and clear message that you've got it all covered. Trust me, this is *not* what you want to convey while caregiving. Instead, it's important to delegate so other people have their own roles. This gives them a chance to feel useful and show love to your person in their own way, and as a result, you will be less depleted and resentful.

Along those lines, I'm not the only one who gets to enjoy Bruce again since he moved into our second home. Now his inner circle has the freedom to step in and take part in his care, too. Before, I thought I was the only one who could do anything for him (have I mentioned that?), and I didn't want to burden anyone. Plus, I'm sure my stress and anxiety didn't exactly set the most inviting tone, making our home feel less like a place where others could comfortably visit and lend a hand. This second home has allowed friends and family members more opportunities to be a part of Bruce's life and care and continue to create their own special memories with him without being micromanaged by me.

For example, a bunch of his guy friends come over weekly, which I know is very meaningful to all of them. I know it is to me. They bring sandwiches and watch whatever game is on TV. Or they sit around, tell stories, and fill the house with love and laughter. "We've got our boys club going," his friend Stephen told me recently. Bruce has always been a guy's guy, and there was truly nothing more important to him than his relationships. The fact that these friendships can continue in this way is exactly what he would want. I love that his friends haven't shied away because of Bruce's health; instead, they have embraced him even more.

If your person moves into a memory care facility, the same can be true for you. It allows your person's friends and family to take part in their care. They can visit freely and create their own traditions without you having to be the gatekeeper and organizer. It also allows you to take a break. Knowing that family or friends are spending time with your person on a given day can offer you the space to step back and recharge, trusting they are in good hands.

## *Your Circle of Support Expands*

After hearing from friends about how beneficial it had been for their loved ones to move into memory care or a skilled nursing home, I've often wondered if we are missing out on the vibrant sense of community these facilities provide, including the other residents, dedicated staff, fellow families, and friends, as well as the various activities that make these places so special. Remember in Chapter 3, I talk about how important and beneficial community is for all of us.

"The obvious benefit of getting help and a memory-care assisted living or skilled nursing facility is you have a respite from the daily, sometimes relentless, activities of caregiving. You have someone to watch your loved one so you can sleep and take care of yourself," explains Katie. "But one thing many of us *don't* realize is that your loved one will have a community to connect with. You may think, 'My loved one can't do anything.' And then you put them in this environment with experts who are trained at engagement and suddenly they're doing things you didn't even know they could."

Katie shared the story of moving her father to memory-care assisted living after seven years of caring for him at home. To her surprise, he got a girlfriend and became in charge of bingo, which gave him purpose, *and* they still spent time together. "It's beautiful to have this whole new world open up, which then just adds more joy and space to everyone's lives," she says.

Another priceless part of this journey is something that I could never have imagined when I resisted getting help: Our care team has become our extended family. There is a special place in heaven for each one of them. The way they look after and love my husband is one of the most beautiful things I have had the privilege to witness. And don't get me started about the puddle I become when I see them lock hands around and with Bruce and pray over him. I can't even write that sentence without crying. I thought no one could care for him like I could; I was so wrong. In fact, they do some things better than I ever could. And as I mentioned, I am his wife once again and our kids get their mom back.

That said, the hard truth about FTD is that some facilities do not accept individuals with this diagnosis. Others may initially allow them to move in but later ask them to leave, realizing they lack the specialized support required. FTD is rarer than Alzheimer's, and many places simply don't have staff trained to manage its unique symptoms and behaviors. Even when facilities believe they can provide care, the complexity and individualized nature of this disease often prove challenging. One of the biggest barriers is the age gap. FTD is the most common form of dementia for people under sixty, while memory care populations are typically much older. This gap in expertise makes some facilities hesitant, concerned they cannot offer the level of care FTD truly demands.

But if your person has FTD, please don't lose hope. There are memory care residences out there that *do* accept individuals with this disease. I've spoken with many FTD care partners who have successfully found the right place for their loved ones, and their stories give me hope. They show that with persistence, the right resources, and a bit of luck, suitable care options are available. This encouragement reminds me that we're not alone in this journey, that there are compassionate people and communities eager to learn how to support those with FTD and you. There are places that can help.

AS TEEPA SAID to me, "We have expectations of care partners that are beyond what they should be, but a single human being can't turn into a superhero. We've got to break the myth that this is normal. It's wrong and it destroys people." I admit that I had expectations of myself that were not realistic, and as a result, I nearly broke trying to attain them. This was bad for me, Bruce, and our children, and if I'd kept going in this manner, I'm not sure I would have been there for my family at all. I could have become part of that statistic of caregivers who die before their person. Bringing in help has also freed up space so I can do things to raise awareness for FTD and support caregivers; for example, without help, I definitely wouldn't have had the bandwidth to be able to write this book or do any advocacy work. Once I let go of perfection-ism and the idea that only I could care for my husband, I not only freed myself up to love Bruce more and care for him better, but I opened *his* world, too. This allowed him to receive attention and love from even more people in his life, including those he'd already had relationships with, like friends and family, and our formal caregivers who have cre-ated their own special bonds with him. It took me a little time to realize this, but if you're able to bring in help, everyone benefits. Because care doesn't diminish when it's shared, it deepens.

## QUESTIONS AND ANSWERS WITH ARLENE SCHOLLAERT

At AFTD's Education Conference in Houston, I attended a session led by social worker Arlene Schollaert and immediately connected with her no-nonsense, direct approach. She didn't sugarcoat the unique and difficult challenges of FTD and pro-vided a clear road map for navigating this journey, emphasizing the importance of seeking help and taking actionable steps to advocate for both yourself and your loved one. Here, Arlene shares why accepting support isn't just beneficial, it's necessary.

**Why is it essential for care partners to acknowledge the impact of their caregiving responsibilities on themselves?**

Caring for someone with FTD or any type of dementia is a marathon not a sprint, so care partners must balance love for their person with self-preservation. That means that you're going to need help and support to remain positive, both physically and emotionally. It happens by integrating services that are going to support you in that process. Whether you're caring for somebody at home or things progress and you need to transition your person to assisted living or memory care, you're still the primary care partner. Your role just changes. So it's really critical to get the pillars of support in place.

### What is the benefit to bringing in help?

- **You improve the quality of your time with your loved one.** When you don't accept help, you can become stressed out, your patience can run thin, and you can become frustrated and short-tempered with your person more frequently. When you start bringing in help, it can improve your relationship with your person, and the time that you spend together can be more quality time.

- **You can sustain yourself on this journey.** It's easy to get isolated from your community, family, and friends when you're caring for someone with FTD or another form of dementia. That isolation can increase stress, anxiety, and depression. It can also cause all sorts of physical symptoms. So it's critical that you seek out a network of support—friends, family, AFTD, support groups, counseling—and get help to improve your emotional and physical well-being. If you don't, it will be very hard to sustain yourself on this journey.

- **You feel more empowered.** There can be a stigma related to having FTD or caring for someone with this or another form of dementia. You may isolate because you're trying to

protect your loved one from exhibiting embarrassing behaviors in public. However, when you do that, you are allowing that stigma to dictate how you manage things. This
takes away your ability to feel empowered because you are
not letting the support in.

- **You become a positive role model.** If you have children,
  which is often the case with early-onset dementia, they are
  watching how you navigate this journey. It's important for
  them to see you taking care of yourself and being able to ask
  for help. This lets them know it's okay to share their feelings
  and ask for help along the way, too.

## Something to think about . . .

What's one small aspect of your life that you can delegate or get help or
support with?

_____

_____

_____

_____

_____

_____

_____

_____

NINE

# Let Friends and Family
# Take Care of You

Nothing changes an opinion quite as powerfully
as when you have an experience.

**KATHLEEN MURPHY, LMFT**

For me, there's nothing more triggering as a caregiver than people saying they have a cure or offering unsolicited advice. It was and still is something I hear over and over again.

*Use coconut oil. Try vigorous exercise, a plant-based diet, no sugar, red light therapy, stem cells. What about B vitamins and lion's mane? Bruce should take saunas, detox from heavy metals, get checked for Lyme disease, sit in an oxygen chamber. What about psilocybin or ayahuasca? Was he on statins?*

These are just some of the numerous comments I hear from people. When I shared the news of Bruce's diagnosis with the public, everyone I knew, and many I didn't, had a cure or an idea for me, something that a friend of a friend of a friend had tried with success. Or, perhaps the worst, they'd say, *I heard there's a new medication for Alzheimer's. Have you tried that?* when that's not even Bruce's diagnosis.

Of course, I know it all comes from a loving and hopeful place. Everyone wants to help. But it is super frustrating and stressful to hear everyone's ideas, especially when you have *already* tried everything in your power to stop or, dare I say, try to reverse the progression of your person's disease. No one considerately and politely asks, "Would you like some suggestions?"

Truthfully, I had tried many things to see if we could "fix" what Bruce had. In the early days before the FTD diagnosis, I directed a lot of energy at reversal and cure, throwing money at various treatments to see what would stick. (Don't underestimate the power and knowledge of a care partner. They are savvy and smart and will try anything and everything within their means and power to change their person's outcome.) With his doctor's approval, I put Bruce through the wringer. Everything we tried was from the lens of "do no harm." You name it, I did it. Each time, my hopes would rise and I'd think, *This is going to be it. THIS is going to turn this "thing" around.* And every time, I was disappointed. Sure, some treatments caused a tiny shift, but it was short-lived. And each time we would try something new, it took years off my life. The planning and organization. Managing and coaching Bruce. It was stressful, to say the least.

Through all that, I was desperate to find the silver bullet so I could yell it from the mountaintops and share it with the world. We were so fortunate we could try different treatments, but none of them worked. In hindsight, some of it felt like snake oil (be aware that some people prey on the sick and their caregivers because we are so sensitive and vulnerable). All it did was leave me feeling deflated, defeated, and even more traumatized.

I don't knock any of the doctors or specialists we saw or treatments we tried. Some of them are beneficial for other diseases. Or they are good for your brain and body but not once you have FTD or any form of dementia. I do believe that prevention is better than cure. Yet none of these "treatments" and no amount of organic coconut oil or lion's mane mushroom was going to help Bruce at the stage we were at. Let's not forget this is a progressive disease. I'm not saying that you shouldn't research, consult with your person's doctor, and perhaps try a variety of things. (When this book comes out, there will probably be more options.) Do so if you have the energy and resources, your loved one is able and willing to participate, and you get the okay from your doctor. Never lose hope. However, that ship has sailed over here. It was time to close that chapter and move forward on our journey knowing I had exhausted all options.

I'm sure you've had people reach out to you with their suggestions as well. If you're open to it, that's wonderful. Yes, they are trying to help and are probably well-meaning. But it may just make you feel worse, at least, that's how I felt. Being a caregiver for a loved one with dementia is hard enough without people weighing in on what they think you should and should not be doing when they don't know the intricacies and inner workings of your person, his or her medical history, your family, and your life.

So how do you deal with unsolicited feedback? How do you know what to take seriously and what to discard? And how can you protect yourself from having to deal with it in the first place? Here are some ideas . . .

## OPINION VS. EXPERIENCE

Everyone will have an opinion, but you have to remind yourself that most don't have the experience to back it up. Hopefully they never will.

And if that's the case, they shouldn't offer their two cents about it and you shouldn't pay them any mind. I learned this from my therapist, Kathleen Murphy.

"Nothing changes an opinion quite as powerfully as when you have an experience," she says. Even if someone is closely familiar with dementia (or the condition you are caregiving for), they aren't in your home, so they don't know how your person is behaving or your family dynamics.

I receive a lot of Instagram comments telling me that I should do things differently. For example, when I took the girls on a vacation last summer and posted photos, people wrote that I should be with my husband. But they're not living my life with my loved one and kids. The vacation offered us a sliver of normalcy and the respite we all needed to recharge. Even though a lot of the opinionated people in your life love you and your person, if they aren't on the front line, day in and day out, you have a choice about whether they get a say. No one else's opinion matters if you don't want it to. Your well-being is what matters.

We have made the choice to put our family's story out there, and with that comes a lot of opinions and criticism. (There has also been so much love and compassion; you can't have one without the other.) Yet it's not always easy to say, "Let them," as I learned from Mel Robbins and mentioned in the last chapter, and let it roll off my back. However, I am working on it and have learned to put my head down and navigate it because I have a mission and purpose. For one, I want to connect with other caregivers in this isolating situation so that they feel seen and supported and so I can as well. The importance of doing that far outweighs some hurtful and misinformed comments from people who don't know me or can't even grasp our situation. I also want to form a larger and meaningful community around myself and our family.

Recently, someone asked me, "Why are you doing all this?" Without hesitation, I answered, "Because I want to live in a world where real treatment options exist, where, one day, FTD comes to an end, and where caregivers are finally seen and supported. My hope is that by lending my voice, our family can be part of the solution."

We all have a role to play. I'm not a doctor or a researcher. I won't be the one running clinical trials or developing the next breakthrough drug. But I can use my voice, my experience, and this book to help make the path a little easier for the next family facing this difficult journey.

Advocacy is how I channel my grief into action. It's how I stand up to FTD by sharing knowledge, building awareness, and supporting other caregivers so they feel less alone. If that helps even one person feel seen or more equipped, then I know I'm doing the work I was meant to do.

## SPEAK UP

What should you do if you're triggered by suggestions or input? Nip it in the bud. Be direct so that people stop sharing their ideas or at least do so in a way that feels better to you. One way to do this is to set appropriate boundaries. This can be hard if you're a people pleaser or worried about hurting other people's feelings, yet it's necessary.

"If people are giving you suggestions, they are being bold, so you are allowed to be bold back," says Kathleen, who helped me, a reformed people pleaser, come up with several ways to respond to these endless recommendations. Tweak the following responses as you see fit, but they're a good start when everyone has an idea for you and you want to defuse the situation and create boundaries:

- "I appreciate your concern; I'll be sure to ask you if I need your advice or suggestions."

- "I know you are trying to help. Thank you. However, when you give advice, it assumes that I have not already done these things and just adds a weight to my shoulders."

- "I appreciate the suggestion, but trying new treatments isn't just about the idea but the cost, time, and logistics, too. Unless there's assistance with those, it can feel more overwhelming than helpful."

- "Thank you for all these suggestions. You might not realize that it's late in the process, so we've already done many of these things."

Also, be up-front with other people about where your loved one is in his or her disease. In the early days, I wanted to throw everything at Bruce's disease to slow its progression and cure it, so I was more open to suggestions. But there comes a point when you can't keep poking and prodding your person anymore or jetting to the other end of the world for the next best thing. Doctors, care teams, and specialists can help guide you in understanding what stage your loved one is in, but often the biggest indicator comes from observing their quality of life. When treatments no longer improve their well-being, or they bring more distress than relief, it may be time to shift the focus from intervention to comfort. You'll know when you've exhausted all options and when both you and your loved one are simply exhausted, too.

## UNDERSTANDING DIFFERENT TYPES OF CARE

As your loved one's needs change, different types of care can help provide the right support at the right time.

- **Supportive care** focuses on managing symptoms and improving daily life while still exploring treatment options. This can include therapies, medications, and lifestyle adjustments.

- **Palliative care** shifts the focus from treatment to comfort and quality of life. It helps ease physical symptoms, reduces stress, and provides emotional support for both the person living with the disease and his or her family. "Meetings are often longer than a traditional physician visit to allow time for the patient and family to speak about concerns. If necessary, caregivers are provided with space for private conversations to discuss issues. Many palliative care programs provide caregiving support and linkage to community programs," says Anne Front, LMFT, an advanced palliative hospice social worker.

- **Hospice care** is a specialized form of palliative care for individuals in the final stage of life. It prioritizes dignity, pain management, and emotional well-being in the time that remains.

"There is a myth that hospice means death or that caregivers are giving up on their loved ones. But placing your loved one in hospice at the right time can give your family the support they need. The idea is to stay one step ahead so your loved one will be provided with comfort care," explains certified dementia practitioner Ty Lewis, who is her mother's caregiver. "Placing my mom in hospice care has given me a fresh perspective on what hospice has to offer at this stage in her care. It has supported us by providing compassionate care, pain management, and in-home support from a doctor, social worker, nurses, and volunteers, and it has allowed me to focus on what matters the most: spending time with her! It gives us time to be present and gives my family a sense of relief knowing all of her care is at home, and I don't have to feel the weight of taking her from place to place while she's in the later stages of her life."

Because these shifts in care can be significant, communication is key. How you choose to communicate is up to you. Some families find it helpful to hold family meetings, in person or on Zoom, to keep everyone on the same page, while others prefer to share updates through email or group messages. What matters most is ensuring that those in your inner circle understand the care plan and feel equipped to offer meaningful support, both to your loved one and to you as the caregiver.

## GIVE YOUR FRIENDS AND FAMILY THE DOS AND DON'TS OF CAREGIVING

Another way to limit suggestions and opinions and get more useful, constructive help from friends and family members is to talk to them. One way to do this is to share the following section with them. You can either hand them this book to read, or take photos of or scan the pages that follow and text them. Not everything will apply to your situation, but my hope is that some of it can help you get the support *you* need.

To the friends and family members of a dementia caregiver:

Thank you for your concern. First, know that your friend or family member is doing one of the hardest jobs ever, one they likely never imagined or prepared for. We know you want to help, but since this is a unique situation, I wanted to share some suggestions, so no one wastes their time and we all benefit. Being a care partner is not something one person can do on his or her own, so your support, no matter how small, can make a world of difference. Your help and concern *is* needed. It's just a matter of what and how.

Here are some dos and don'ts I've gathered from my own experience and that of other care partners I've spoken to:

*Do* have compassion. There is a common misconception that caregivers have it figured out—they've got it covered and they are good. In most cases, that's simply not true. Caregivers are often thrown into this role with no training and no experience. Imagine taking *any* job with no experience. This is the same thing, but often caregivers don't have a choice about whether to take the job or not, and they don't have time to get educated beforehand.

*Do* tell the care partner what a good job they are doing. Care partners are unsung heroes who often don't get any praise.

*Do* call just to check in. Care partners spend long hours with their person who has dementia, which means that real, adult conversations may be minimal to nonexistent.

*Do* research the specific dementia they are caregiving for. This shows that you care, builds trust, and helps you ask more thoughtful questions. For example, not all dementias affect memory, so asking, "Does your person still know who you are?" might be frustrating. Caregivers are already exhausted from explaining their situations. Doing some research beforehand makes conversations more meaningful and helps them feel seen and supported.

*Do* ask how the care partner is doing, too. Most people ask how the person with dementia is doing, but with many forms of dementia, it's harder on the care partner. Please don't forget about them.

*Do* ask if they feel comfortable sharing what treatments and medications they have tried, but do so with curiosity and care, not judgment. And make it clear that it's okay if they do not want to reveal this information because it is very personal.

*Do* know your audience. The person you're speaking to has likely tried countless things and may feel discouraged, sensitive, or frustrated that nothing has made a significant difference. While your suggestions come from a place of love, the care partner might not be able to receive them that way, especially if they're overwhelmed or exhausted. A little empathy and timing can go a long way. Sometimes, just being present and listening is the most helpful thing you can offer.

If you bring in a suggestion, *do* the legwork for it, such as research and possibly even arranging the treatment and payments. The care partner may not take you up on this, but at least you're not just dropping a suggestion, which can feel like another item on the care partner's already overwhelming to-do list.

*Do* offer specific ways to help rather than saying, "Let me know if you need anything." Most caregivers aren't going to reach out when they need help, either because they feel shame, they don't want to be a burden, they think they can do everything on their own, or they don't even know what they need help with because it's too overwhelming to even think about. Instead, think about all the things you do for yourself. Chances are it's similar to what the care partner needs to do, too, but doesn't have the time or energy. Here are some suggestions for how you can help:

- **Ask if the caregiver has the right mental health support in place.** If they don't, help the caregiver find it. This might mean locating a support group, therapist, and/or a way to schedule in some time for themselves. If the caregiver has children, ask if the children need support and/or help research it.

- **Offer to stay with the care partner's person so they can have a break.** This allows the caregiver to do things alone or with their children or other loved ones. There may be a time that is least taxing, like when the person sleeps.

- **If the caregiver has children of his or her own, offer to drive them to activities, take them to school, or help with homework.** FTD in particular strikes much younger people who often have kids going through their own milestone moments, like applying to college or learning to drive. Perhaps you can offer to help with applications, school tours, driving lessons, or school pickups and drop-offs.

- **Knock things off the care partner's overwhelming to-do list** by picking up prescriptions, calling to make medical appointments (for the patient but also annual visits for the care partner), doing laundry, cleaning their house, or getting their car serviced or washed.

- **Stop by in the morning and have a cup of coffee with them so they feel less isolated.** Just call or text first to make sure it's a good time.

- **Drive the care partner and their person to and from an appointment.** Be their curbside driver so they don't have to deal with parking and the dreaded parking structure.

- **Offer to go to doctors' appointments,** especially the big ones where the care partner is receiving a lot of new information. They are often so overwhelmed that it's helpful to have someone else in the room to listen and take notes or record the meeting.

- **If they have children, take their kids out to dinner or a movie.**

- **Clean out all the processed foods in their kitchen and refill the fridge and pantry with brain-healthy options** like those mentioned in Chapter 5. Of course, get the caregiver's permission first.

- **Give them a gift card to a delivery service** like DoorDash, Postmates, or Grubhub, or a housecleaning service.

- **Reach out to the care partner's network of friends and family members.** You can create a schedule to bring meals to the family or a list of tasks that the care partner's community can sign up for. There are so many apps and websites that make it easy to do this.

- **Encourage the caregiver to create a list of all the tasks they do for their person and the rest of their family—** such as make dinner, mow the lawn, or return library books—or offer to make the list for them. Then have them refer to the list when you want to help.

- **Start a GoFundMe page.** Ask the caregiver if you can raise funds to help them pay for things like a nighttime caregiver or respite care.

*Do* remember it's all about support. This is not a solo mission. Care partners need help to stay both physically and emotionally healthy but are often unable to ask for it or don't even know they need it. What you offer may not fix everything, but showing up in thoughtful, consistent ways can make a real difference.

*Don't* offer unsolicited advice when possible. Caregiving is deeply personal, and no two experiences are the same. Even if you've been a caregiver, factors like family dynamics and symptoms differ. While sharing advice may seem helpful, too much input can feel overwhelming. Caregivers already question if they're doing enough; outside opinions can add pressure. Instead, ask: "Would you like a suggestion?" This keeps the conversation supportive and respectful. Also, sometimes it helps just to listen rather than try to offer advice or problem-solve.

*Don't* mention new treatments, trials, or medications you've heard about, especially if you're not certain the person has that specific condition. Most care partners are already working closely with neurologists or doctors who can point them in the right direction.

That said, *how* you bring something up can make all the difference. If you feel like you have something worth sharing, say it gently. You might start with: "I'm not sure if you've already heard of this, but I wanted to pass it along just in case . . ." Then offer what you've found. If you can, provide a pamphlet or a one-page summary so the caregiver can look it over at his or her own pace, without feeling put on the spot.

If you are going to offer advice, *don't* say, "You should try ____." This makes me wonder, *What do you think I've been doing all this time? Twiddling my thumbs?* Instead, preface a suggestion with "Is ___ something that you've thought of?" or "You probably already looked into this, but on the off chance you didn't, have you heard about ___?" This feels more respectful of everything the care partner has been through. The bottom line is that many caregivers are in a fragile and sensitive state, so be gentle with your approach because they really wish their person was not ill.

After a visit with their person, *don't* tell the care partner, "He seems fine." Keep in mind you are getting a small slice of time in a twenty-four-hour period. Even if the person does seem "fine" or "better" during your visit, that's not indicative of what the care partner is regularly dealing with and can be irritating and triggering to hear. *Do* tell the care partner that they are doing a beautiful job under difficult circumstances.

*Don't* say, "You've got this." It can feel dismissive, because honestly, I don't always feel like I do. Instead, what truly helps is hearing "I'm here for you, no matter what," "You're not alone in this," and "I know this isn't easy, but you're showing up with so much strength and love."

*Don't* give up. The care partner in your life may say no to invitations for coffee, walks, visits, etc. because they're so overwhelmed. After a while, some people stop asking. But eventually, care partners want and need those invitations, so even if your offer gets declined, keep asking. Care partners still appreciate feeling included and remembered.

## REACHING OUT MADE EASY

One idea is to send the caregiver in your life a specific list of things you can do for them. Not only is this thoughtful, it's an easy and lighthearted way to remove his or her feelings of being a burden. For example, you can send a text or email that is something like this:

Hi there. I'm just checking in. I'm free to help out this week so would love for you to choose from the following:

1. I can run errands for you on any day after 2:00 p.m. I can drop items right at your door—no need to even greet me or have a conversation if you're not up for it.

2. I can take your kids out to dinner on Wednesday, Thursday, or Friday. Of course, we will bring you back something delicious to eat, too.

3. I can have dinner from a restaurant of your choice sent to you and your family.

It's okay if you don't need or want any of the above right now. Just know that I'm sending you loving thoughts and, if it's okay with you, I can revisit this list with you in a week or so. I want you to know I'm here for you.

"Sometimes friends stop reaching out
because they don't know what to say or they
don't know what do. But sometimes it's not about
any of that, it's simply about being a friend."

ARLENE SCHOLLAERT,
*LCSW, family services director of*
*Amazing Place, Houston, Texas*

BY THIS POINT in the book, you know that caregiving is not a solo journey and that it's okay and necessary for you to reach out for help. Those in your inner circle want to support you; in fact, it makes them feel connected to your loved one and gives them a sense of purpose and, as I mentioned earlier in the book, can create a closer bond between you and that person. While it might feel strange to hand someone this chapter, remember that those who care about you and your loved one want to do and say the right things. Sharing this can empower them with thoughtful language that avoids triggers, as well as practical ideas for how they can step in and provide meaningful support. Navigating this journey is hard for you and for those around you who aren't sure what to say or how to help. By educating them, you're not only giving them tools to help in your situation, you're equipping them to better support others they may encounter on a similar path. And one day, if they find themselves in the caregiving boat, you'll already be speaking the same language.

*Something to think about . . .*

The next time someone offers unsolicited advice, what is one thing you can say to yourself, to the other person, or both?

_____

_____

_____

_____

_____

_____

_____

_____

_____

_____

_____

_____

_____

_____

_____

_____

_____

_____

_____

What are some supportive things that someone else could do for you?

_____

_____

_____

_____

_____

_____

_____

_____

_____

_____

_____

_____

_____

_____

_____

_____

_____

_____

# TEN

# Reframe the Journey

*If you look for new hope and purpose in the midst of dealing with something terrible, it can lighten your load.*

**DR. PAULINE BOSS,**
*author of* Loving Someone
Who Has Dementia

Sometimes people see my social media and think that I'm okay or say that I seem so strong. "I don't know how you do it," they tell me. But you know what? I'm not okay. I'm really not. And I'm not always strong. Watching someone you love lose pieces of themselves is incredibly painful and traumatic, especially someone like Bruce, who was so capable, smart, and high-functioning, and who cherished his life to the fullest. FTD is deeply unkind. It's a beast of a disease, and for Bruce, the progression has been slow every step of the way. All I can do is shake my head and remain "befuddled," as he used to say. *Why him? How could this happen?* What a great loss for us all.

My grief about this can still paralyze me. It's always at the surface. I still cry. I'm still shocked and remain in disbelief at this disease and at the turn our lives have taken and the things we've lost. I've noticed that sometimes I walk around with my shoulders slumped and the spring in my step is gone. I still have a hard time accepting what is, yet FTD doesn't give you many options. It can suck all the air out of a room. So I've made a choice to pump oxygen back into our lives, for the sake of our girls, Bruce, and me. And to give the middle finger to this disease.

When Bruce was first diagnosed, I was angry. I wasted precious energy fighting it and fighting it and fighting it. But the more you fight it, the harder it is, and I know who wins in the end: the disease. No matter what you do, you can't stop its progression. You can throw all the money you want at it, but it's not stopping—been there, done that. You can put all your energy into it, and it's not stopping—been there, done that, too.

Then I woke up one day and thought, I don't have a choice about Bruce having this disease, but I do have a choice in terms of how I react. I can wallow in sorrow, or I can take some power back and make the best of it for all of us. I can focus on what we have lost, or I can focus on how much I have gained, this beautiful caregiving community, and what we still have to celebrate, like our two bright, fun, and healthy daughters and a larger family unit built on mutual respect and admiration. I can let waves of negativity, doom, and constant dread weigh me down, or I can strive for peace.

I call this the remarkable reframe. Even though there is immense sadness and deep grief, I am choosing to shift my perspective. To survive this, I have to find meaning in the pain and channel it into something purposeful. I need to turn my grief into action and create good from something so profoundly difficult. I need to find joy. I have a calling and need to help others. I know Bruce would want me to do that, and I know my girls need to see that. Standing up to FTD in this way has been empowering and healing to a certain degree. We only get one life, and we can't allow this disease to take all of it.

Look, as caregivers, we don't have much agency in terms of when or how dementia comes into our lives, but we have agency in terms of which lens we view it through. We can choose to be angry, sad, and in our grief all the time (and trust me, there are days when that's *exactly* what I feel like doing). Or we can break up our doom-and-gloom thinking. Yes, caregiving is hard, stressful, and scary. Yes, we are alone in so much of what we do day by day, hour by hour. But reframing this journey can make it a little lighter and brighter, especially if you have children or other people traveling it with you.

This remarkable reframe isn't about just thinking positively, and I hope it doesn't come across as toxic positivity because I don't subscribe to that—especially on this serious and heavy road as a caregiver. For me, it's a way of looking at this caregiving journey that feels empowering, one that makes space for the hard stuff but also leaves room for the moments of meaning and connection that can come from this experience. As we learned earlier, it's something Dr. Pauline Boss calls "both/and" thinking. Both can and do exist: the sadness and constant grief, as well as the beauty that unfolds. We can choose to make this journey horrific and terrible, which it is, *and* it can also be joyous, and there can be happiness and laughter. And if you're like me and have children, nieces, nephews, or other young people watching you navigate this rough path, it's important to model the ability to reframe *any* obstacle that comes your way.

This isn't the life I imagined, and it's not what I'd choose for us. But this is what has been presented to our family, and I have dedicated myself to walking Bruce and our young girls through it the best way that I can. I'm learning how to live alongside FTD, which is truly a balancing act.

Look, I know it's not always easy to do this. The tunnel can feel very dark, lonely, and scary. I know that because I have been there. I'm still there. But there are cracks of light along the way that I can't ignore, and because I have faith in the process, I trust there is something bright and glorious at the end. So I'll keep walking toward it. I need to, in order to show up for our two daughters in the healthiest way and honor my husband and myself while I'm on this earth.

And let me acknowledge this: You might not be at the point where you can reframe this journey yet. If that's the case, I get it. Honestly, there was a time during this experience when I would not have been ready to hear about reframing either. But my hope is that you will be able to revisit this chapter in time when you're ready. I never thought I'd be here, but I am. And although it's not a straight line, and there are days when I'm still pissed and unable to reframe, it does get better.

Here are some ways I think about reframing our journey, and that I use to make this unchosen path feel less dark and more purposeful. Perhaps they can help you, too.

## REMARKABLE REFRAME: I CAN DECIDE TO ACCEPT MY LOVED ONE'S DISEASE

In addition to teaching me about both/and thinking, Dr. Boss taught me about the need for acceptance. Acceptance, as she describes it, doesn't mean giving up or being okay with the situation. Instead, it means acknowledging reality as it is, without denial or resistance, and finding ways to live alongside it. It's about letting go of what you can't control while focusing on what you can.

When we talked about acceptance, Dr. Boss explained that instead of using the word "acceptance" she prefers to say, "I've *decided* to accept."

"I'm not terribly fond of the word 'acceptance' because it means you have to surrender," she says. "I prefer you say, 'I've decided to accept,' which means *you* have more agency because it was your decision." This is especially important because caregivers are caught in a situation that is mostly outside of our control, so anyplace we can feel like *we* are making a choice is beneficial. For this reason, I decided to accept FTD and the ambiguity that it causes.

"This [acceptance] is crucial because, for many people, the disease is going to go on for a long time, and you have to stay strong in order to bear the ambiguity of 'he's here and he's also not here,'" says Dr. Boss.

For me, deciding to accept FTD has been both freeing and stabilizing. I'm no longer fighting against what is, which only kept me stuck and prevented me from moving forward. I'm no longer in denial. Instead, I'm working to embrace this journey. If it feels right for you, or when you are ready, try saying to yourself, "I've decided to accept this journey." Take a moment to notice how it feels in your mind and body. Do you feel your muscles loosening and gripping less tightly? (We don't realize how much tension we hold in our bodies.) Does it take the edge off? You might even begin to cry. Saying this might not work for everyone, but I'll admit it has done wonders for me and it's worth giving it a shot.

## REMARKABLE REFRAME:
## I CAN FIND JOY IN THE LITTLE THINGS

As Bruce's disease progressed, I had so much distress around whether it was okay for me to do anything for myself when my husband was living with FTD. And I'm talking about something as small as walking in a nearby park or getting a cup of coffee with a friend. It took some time and a lot of therapy, but eventually I realized that it's okay for me to live, and that me living didn't take anything away from Bruce. What I noticed in this process, as my family's life was being stripped away, was that I love life. In fact, I didn't know how much I loved it until things unraveled. I realized there are very small moments that we take for granted, like enjoying the scenic route home or stopping for an iced coffee without a care in the world.

As you know, the role of dementia caregiver doesn't just happen one day. It's a slow burn, and looking back, it can be hard to see where your role as child/spouse/partner/fill-in-the-blank morphed into that of caregiver. In that blurry process, I stepped out of my life and onto the sidelines. Part of my reframe was realizing that this needed to change. I didn't want to just survive amid the sadness. I wanted to thrive, and as I've mentioned, I learned that thriving doesn't mean Bruce is any worse off and me *not* thriving won't make him better.

Because of this disease, the littlest things bring me so much more joy than they used to. For example, since I was able to put the right support in place, I can now relish something as simple as picking the girls up at school on a Friday and spontaneously saying, "Let's go get dinner and ice cream at the mall." I appreciate it ten times more than I did pre-

FTD. That's the reframe. I make a conscious effort every morning when I open my eyes to connect to gratitude and think about how I can make that day rewarding. I do that for myself, and I do that for our two children. I also do it for Bruce, who would not want it any other way for me. I'm certain that if roles were reversed, Bruce would be doing the same; after all, as I've shared previously, one of his favorite sayings was "live it up," and I would want him to make beautiful memories with our girls, not spend his days angry, resentful, and on edge, which would negatively affect them. I want to honor him and teach my girls to do the same. That's also the reframe.

"You get to live. You get to be interested in things, and you don't have to sacrifice your life because your loved one is sick," my therapist, Kathleen, told me, and still reminds me. It's very easy for me to fall back into wanting to isolate and decline invitations from friends or family. But I don't want to take any more joy away from my kids. They have been through a lot with their dad, and there is so much they have lost. Despite that, I want them to enjoy their childhood, not to look back and see it completely clouded by FTD.

Getting here was a long process and it did not come easily, and yes, we hit bumps along the way. But I make it a conscious effort. Finding small pockets of joy where I can helps; perhaps looking at life this way can help you, too. So, what moments bring you even a tiny sense of joy? Is it listening to your favorite song, taking a walk in nature, or sharing a laugh with a friend? Could you plan something small, like a coffee date, a quick dance break, or a quiet moment to read? Think about where you can create space, even just a sliver, for something that feels good in your day. It may seem hard to do at first, but those moments can make all the difference.

## REMARKABLE REFRAME:
## I LIVE IN THE HERE AND NOW

One lesson I've learned on this unexpected journey is the importance of being in the here and now, not putting off until tomorrow what I can do today, and continuing to work toward personal goals that can get hijacked during the caregiving journey. I've realized that caregiving is just a role in my life, a big role, but it does not define me, and it's not my whole being. I'm trying to be more present with the girls and more spontaneous overall, something Bruce taught me.

You can't control everything. And I'm saying that from a place of having driven myself crazy trying to do and control everything. It didn't work. It just made me crazier, made my energy negative, and made me lose patience with everyone around me. Things are going to happen. That's a given with this disease. You can't prepare for everything, but you can choose to embrace the new world that you are living in.

For me, as with many things, this is a work in progress. For example, it's not easy to make new memories without Bruce and do things with the girls that he and I talked about experiencing as a family. But it is Bruce who motivates me to do just that. As I've mentioned, he was fun and wanted everyone around him to have fun, too, so that's the way our family will keep honoring him.

With this in mind, I decided to take Mabel and Evelyn on one of the trips Bruce and I dreamed of doing with them: Japan in the spring to see the cherry blossoms. (Full-circle moment: In my late teens I flew to Japan on a modeling contract. Those were the days when everyone on the plane watched the same movie that was being shown on a small TV high up along the aisle, and *Armageddon* was playing. Tears streamed down my face as I watched Bruce's character say goodbye to his daughter, played by Liv Tyler.)

Our trip to Japan was so meaningful—after all, the girls were at an age where they could appreciate the food and culture—but it was also heartbreaking to do it without Bruce. I tried to be mindful and not bring the mood down by saying, "If Dad was here, he would have said this" or "Gosh, your dad would have loved that," but that doesn't mean I didn't think those things. Often. Because he would have cherished every moment of that trip. Just writing this brings tears to my eyes for him, me, and our whole family. But as we say in the FTD community, "It is what it is," and to honor Bruce, I have to reframe this journey and hold gratitude as well as grief. (This is part of the both/and thinking we've talked about.)

Another thing that helps is the mantra my therapist, Kathleen, taught me: "Stay here, don't go there." Saying this out loud brings me back to the present and helps me stop worrying about future what-ifs. I might have to repeat it to myself twenty times a day, but it works. I start to feel my feet beneath me, connect back into my body, and slow my breathing down. Say it with me: "Stay here, don't go there." Try this when you feel your thoughts getting too far ahead of you and you need to bring yourself back to the here and now. It can also help to write it on a Post-it note and hang it where you can see it, or set it as a reminder that pops up regularly on your phone.

## REMARKABLE REFRAME:
## MY PERSON IS STILL HERE

FTD is awful, and it's traumatic to watch it slowly steal your person. Other forms of dementia are tragic as well. But here's the reframe: These diseases give you time with the person you love.

They aren't taken right there and then.

"The long goodbye of Alzheimer's can be looked at as a gift when compared to sudden and brutal deaths in other tragedies," says Patti Davis. When she and I talked about this, we reflected on how unpredictable life is, how people can leave us in an instant, sometimes without the chance to even say goodbye. As heartbreaking as dementia is, it offers something rare: time. Time to sit together, to express love, and to cherish even the smallest moments. It's not the path any of us would choose, but there's beauty in the quiet opportunities it gives us to connect while we can.

With dementia, you're not with the person you once knew, but you can be with a new version of the person you're caring for. I know this can be hard. For me, there are rare moments when the old Bruce emerges in that smirk, twinkle, smile, or gesture that makes me laugh like I used to. Those glimmers take me back in time. Yet as quickly as they come, they go, and when I am thrust back into reality with a jolt, I'm met with intense grief and unbearable sadness. Sometimes I think I'd prefer not to see those glimmers at all and instead embrace this new person. But those moments also remind me that Bruce is still here, and ultimately, I'm grateful for every glimpse of him, no matter how brief or how painful it might be for me.

Remind yourself that at least some part of your loved one is still with you, even if it's not the same relationship or person you've always known. So if you have those fleeting moments, too, as hard as they might be, take a second to appreciate them. That's the reframe. The choice I make is to accept that there is good that comes with the bad.

I'm trying to teach this to my girls, too. It's painful for them to see their dad as he is today and, because they're so young, these seem to be their most vivid memories of him right now. That's the bad. The good is that they still have time with him, and as a result, they have been able to slowly settle into the idea of his disease and gracefully and beautifully meet him where he is.

Another part of the reframe is that they get to see that we're surrounding their dad with so much love and care, and they're learning that this is what we do for the people we hold dear. They get to watch other family members and friends continue to show up for Bruce. I hope this shows them how much their dad meant to so many people, both within our intimate circle and beyond it, and how important relationships were to Bruce. I hope it shows them how blessed and fortunate we are, because even though this is terrible, it could always be worse. That isn't just the reframe—that is what I know to be true.

## REMARKABLE REFRAME:
## MY PERSON IS LIVING IN THE PRESENT

Yes, it's hard to see what FTD has done to someone who was so vibrant, funny, wild, and caring. But when I look at Bruce now, he's quite blissful. He's not thinking about what happened yesterday or what's happening in an hour. He's in the here and now and very present. He's not in pain. It's one of the most beautiful things to witness. (As a worrier with a mind that is constantly spinning, I sometimes wonder what that must be like.)

Of course, it's not ideal, but that's the reframe. That's how you find beauty in the sadness. Bruce's disease, I believe, has given him this one grace: to not know what FTD is. This might be the only thing I appreciate about it. If Bruce had said, "Emma, I think something's wrong with me. I'm scared," it would have been deeply distressing to me. I'm grateful that I did not have that experience. Instead, I think about something Bruce said often: "I'm just a regular guy who has had an incredibly blessed life."

That can be your reframe, too. If your person is not aware of what is unfolding, see it as a blessing that they are not scared or worried. They are just living minute by minute, surrounded by your care and love.

## REMARKABLE REFRAME: CAREGIVING IS TRANSFORMATIVE

Even amid the grief, trauma, and immense sadness, becoming Bruce's care partner has been one of the most rewarding and transformative experiences of my life. It has reshaped who I am at a cellular level, for the better. I've become more compassionate. I'm able to hold more space, patience, and understanding for what others might be going through. I have more confidence in myself and my abilities, which has been invaluable. By no means is this journey easy, nor am I doing it perfectly—I've made plenty of mistakes and no doubt will make more, but I've chosen to grow from each one. I figured that if this was going to be our new life, I wanted to make the very most of it.

But I didn't arrive at this perspective overnight. In those early days, I felt far from it, which is why I'm glad this book is in your hands now. When we first received the diagnosis, everything felt heavy and overwhelming. Even before that, when I didn't yet know what was wrong, I had to step up, balancing Bruce's care with that of our girls.

As a parent, your instinct is always to put your children first. But there were times when prioritizing Bruce's well-being was necessary because his stability allowed everything in our home to function more smoothly. It was a delicate balancing act, one that didn't always feel clear or easy, but looking back, I'm proud of how far I've come. I've gained a deeper understanding of caregiving, this disease, and how to advocate not just for Bruce, but for myself and my family. More than anything, I'm proud of how much I've grown as a person. This journey has profoundly shaped how I see the world.

Along the way, applaud yourself for the work you're doing, truly one of the hardest jobs in the world, and take note of how you have grown. Stop to acknowledge the things that you are learning and new skills that you're adopting. This is no small feat.

## REMARKABLE REFRAME: I AM EXPERIENCING UNCONDITIONAL LOVE

My connection to Bruce now is different than when we started, but it's also so much deeper. Although it's hard to articulate this, let me try. First, it's beautiful to know and feel this kind of unconditional love and appreciation for my husband. Like the love a parent has for their children, it comes with no expectations. What I've realized is that prior to FTD, my relationship with Bruce had conditions—many conditions, in fact. I expected him to be my partner in every sense: to help plan for our future, be present and emotionally available not just for me but for all our children, and meet my needs in specific ways.

Before I knew that Bruce's brain was slowly changing thanks to FTD, we went through a period where we struggled with a lot of miscommunications and an inability to connect, something so painful to me since we'd always seemed in sync. I felt like I was banging my head against a brick wall and was often frustrated and confused. We didn't seem aligned on our plans for the future anymore, our traditions seemed to be falling by the wayside, and our shared responsibilities became anything but, well, shared. All of this made me contemplate divorce.

When I realized that the changes in Bruce were caused by something beyond his control, I softened quickly. I then understood that the kind, caring, and compassionate man I fell in love with was there the whole time. It was his *disease* that had started to take away the traits that made him *him*. I was able to forgive and forget, and I fell back in love with Bruce in a different, reimagined, and unconditional way. What a gift that is, especially because I'd spent my whole life wanting to know and feel unconditional love with a partner.

Growing up, we didn't live in one place for an extended period of time. When my parents were married, my dad's job at an American oil company took us all over the world. I was born in Malta, and then we lived in Lebanon, Saudi Arabia, Venezuela, and Texas, to name just a few, until we settled in California when I was seven and my parents divorced. From there, my mom and I moved to Tottenham in London. With this constant change, nothing felt normal or secure. This is not a criticism of my mother, because she was my safety and felt like home no matter where we were, but the things happening around us felt uncertain and a little chaotic at times. I yearned for stability. I wanted a home where you planted roots and made lasting memories. So as immature as this may sound, I longed for the fairy-tale romance that I saw in the movies. A calm, "normal" life with the white picket fence really appealed to me, as did a relationship built on unconditional love. This disease has brought that kind of love; it's not the way I wanted to experience it, but I did get what I asked for and try to see that as a blessing.

Part of this is that my expectations have softened, too. Before Bruce's disease, he always made occasions like anniversaries and birthdays very extra. For example, he'd send me dozens and dozens of roses. (Although I love flowers, I could never bring myself to tell him I don't actually love roses because his intention was so sweet.) Or he'd make a dinner reservation at my favorite restaurant and order a beautiful bottle of Cabernet because he knew I didn't like champagne. I loved how Bruce celebrated everything in such a big way; for example, your birthday wasn't just celebrated on the actual *day*, it was birthday *month*. It was wild and fun and a world I didn't know before him. The difficult part was that he set the bar high for himself, so as his disease progressed, he couldn't keep up with it, and this was confusing and sad for me. Especially as he was the romantic in our relationship. Now when our anniversary or my birthday rolls around, I no longer have the anticipation of what may happen. But the beauty of that is, we just get to be. I can sit with Bruce and appreciate the life and family we have created and tried to maintain. Yes, I mourn what was, but I also feel so grateful to experience a love that is limitless and comes with no expectations.

If you're taking care of a loved one—a partner, a parent, a friend, even a child—you're practicing something many of us talk about but few of us truly get to put into action: unconditional love. You're looking after your person's needs without expectation, without conditions. That is no small thing. Take a moment to recognize what that means. The energy and care you're giving come from a place of pure love and connection. And while it can feel exhausting, it's also profoundly beautiful. In practicing this, you're not only caring for your person, you're embodying a love that will nourish and transform you. So when it feels overwhelming, remember this: You are showing up in the purest, most meaningful way possible. And that is an incredible gift, not just for them, but for you, too.

## REMARKABLE REFRAME:
## MY PERSON HAS TAUGHT ME SO MUCH

"We tend to ask, 'Why? Why did my loved one get Alzheimer's when that really mean guy down the block is fine? Why didn't he get it?'" says Patti. "Although it's human and natural to ask why, it's the wrong question. You'll never understand why, so don't waste your time there. Better questions are 'What can I learn from this?' and 'How can I grow from this experience?' If you're open to whatever lessons are folded into this situation, then you can change your experience of the experience, at least in small ways."

There's so much I learned from Bruce that has helped me on this journey. As I mentioned, being raised by a single mom who did it all herself, I was taught to be independent and self-reliant. So I was grateful when Bruce walked into my world, because he took the reins. I could finally relax and let down my guard. I learned from his confidence and take-charge manner. I was so comfortable standing next to him, even a little behind him, to be honest, and now I have to lead him and our family. It was scary at first, *so* scary. Bruce's world is huge, but because of what he taught me about leading, I now do it with great pride. I feel like I'm passing what he taught me to our girls, helping them become resilient and capable, something that would make him so proud and happy. (After all, Bruce always said, "Women should be in charge of everything—they should be the presidents of every country in the world. Guys can't compete; they just kind of run through life messing things up.")

I'm also grateful for all I've learned from Bruce throughout his journey with FTD. He has brought more love, compassion, and empathy into our world. Learning how to support him and our young family has empowered me in many ways. I've become a problem solver, a doer, and very capable. These are parts of my personality and character I didn't know existed, or at least not to this extent. No, I don't have it down to a science, especially because things are forever changing as Bruce's disease progresses and our girls get older, yet I'm always learning and growing. And it's the confidence Bruce exuded that I grabbed on to, which helps me do this each and every day.

When you have a minute, write down a few things *you* have learned on this journey, or skills you've gained that you had no idea you could possess. Keep this list close by and add to it as time goes on. Look at it when you need a reframe or a moment to pat yourself on the back.

## REMARKABLE REFRAME: MY FAMILY IS LEARNING, TOO

The other day, I was taking Mabel to a doctor's appointment and this woman in the car ahead of us pulled right in front of the medical building in a no-parking zone. I was frustrated, unsure I could drive around her since there was just a sliver of a space next to her car.

"What is this person doing?" I huffed. "Why are they stopping right there?"

"Mom, maybe it's a caregiver trying to get their person with dementia out of the car," Mabel said. "Just wait."

Wow. She was so right. While I could have had more patience with the person parking in the wrong spot, Mabel had so much empathy and a different way of thinking. Is that from her experience with Bruce? I think so. This is a part of the fabric of who both of my girls are. They are kind, caring, and thoughtful young ladies navigating their new reality with beauty and total grace, and continuing to teach me a thing or two in the midst of it.

When Evelyn was in fourth grade, she came home from school and said to me, "Did you know that people with dementia can become severely dehydrated?"

"No, I didn't," I replied. "How did you learn that?" She went on to explain that she had some free time at school, so she decided to look up "fun facts" about dementia.

Now, we all know dementia isn't exactly "fun," but she was only eight or nine at the time, and I have to admit, it made me chuckle. She's definitely her father's child, curious and always eager to learn and share random "fun" facts.

"Thank you for letting me know," I told her. "We'll always make sure that Daddy has a bottle of water nearby."

Then I went on to tell her, "What you just did is one of the most loving and compassionate things you can do for someone you care about. Staying curious and educating yourself about what they're going through and how to best support them is a true act of love and kindness."

You're not the only one learning on this caregiving journey. Everyone in your inner circle—children, nieces and nephews, parents, close friends—is being changed by this experience. Our girls have had to grow up more quickly and witness more than they should have to at their ages. It makes me sad to see some of their innocence taken away, and there are parts of it I can't control, so, like so much of the FTD journey, I have decided to accept it. They've had a lot to process and lost so much throughout this traumatic, heartbreaking turn of events, and yet it could have been worse. After all, they have witnessed what love is and how we show up for the people who matter most. It's changed who they are for the better. I am so proud of these two young ladies.

Shortly after Bruce's diagnosis, I was talking about the girls to our close family friend Robert Kraft. He said, "These are the cards your kids have been dealt, and they will learn to play them."

This quote has stuck with me ever since. Yes, they have been dealt some shitty cards, but they play them with skill and will continue to do so.

## REMARKABLE REFRAME:
## I'M MAKING AN IMPACT ON MY PERSON

I hope it brings you solace to know that what you are doing is noble and admirable. This is especially the case if you're caring for someone you're not close to or have a difficult relationship with, which comes with its own set of complications.

Giving back to Bruce has given me a sense of self-worth. One day, I will leave this earth knowing that I made a positive impact on someone's life when I knew, inevitably, his disease would win in the end. I work hard to ensure that Bruce is comfortable and cared for in the best way. In fact, I am proud of myself for how I have been able to handle this disease on his behalf.

I always hear people say, "I don't know how you do it. I couldn't do it." But I think they are selling themselves short; most people would show up and that's the beauty of humanity, because there is no other way around this disease but through it. No one wants to have to walk this journey, but when it knocks, they will answer the door, just like *you* are doing.

It's rewarding to learn how to care for Bruce and gain new life skills. It's not something I would have ever fathomed, but I celebrate the way I've been able to show up for him and our family. I'd like to think he'd be proud, too.

I'd like you to take a moment to acknowledge yourself here. I know how hard it is to pat ourselves on the back, so if you can't say this about yourself, I will. I'm very proud of you. And Bruce would tell you, "You're doing great."

## TALK KINDLY TO YOURSELF

One important reframe for us as caregivers is how we talk to ourselves. I know I often beat myself up, saying things like, "I didn't have enough patience today" or "Emma, what's the matter with you?" My therapist, Kathleen, taught me how to change this.

"Instead of being hard on yourself, compliment yourself with an affectionate internal voice," she explains. For example, on days when I don't have patience, I reframe and soften that inner voice by telling myself, "Okay, it wasn't a great afternoon. But tomorrow's a new day," or "That was a difficult day, but you sure did show up." It's so easy to talk badly to ourselves. Please try to shift that inner voice. Give yourself some compassion and understand that what you are doing is hard.

## REMARKABLE REFRAME: I CAN BRING MY LOVED ONE INTO THE BIG MOMENTS

Recently, Mabel graduated from sixth grade. It's always tough when these milestones happen because Bruce can't attend. Under different circumstances, Bruce wouldn't have missed a thing, since he loved nothing more than to root his girls on. In fact, I can say with confidence that his would have been the loudest "WOO!" in the room, the kind that would probably embarrass a twelve-year-old immensely! But when people say their loved one is there in spirit, I believe it. So as nuts as this may sound, at these events I close my eyes and channel Bruce into the moment. I intentionally tap into his subconscious and bring him in.

Listen, we are living in a way that feels unconventional from morning to night. Nothing about this journey feels "normal." Channeling him into the moment brings me some peace and settles my sadness. So do whatever helps you honor your feelings and your loved one when they can't participate in life's biggest or smallest moments.

If this sounds too woo-woo for you, try carrying one of your person's belongings, something that fits in your pocket or that you can hold or touch that connects you to them. Bruce was a handkerchief kind of guy, so I always have one of his in my pocket or bag. It's another way to bring him to these meaningful affairs, and with all the tears I shed at these events, I end up using it anyway.

These days, when my mom and I watch the girls do their thing, sometimes joined by other family members who come along to cheer them on, we beam at them with pride. As we did at Mabel's graduation, we also cry tears of happiness for their accomplishments, as well as tears of sadness that their dad can't be there. Without fail, my mom will lean over and say, "Bruce would have loved this." This is something I always think about in those moments but don't have the strength to utter out loud, as I would break down. I'm happy my mom can verbalize and acknowledge what I'm thinking.

## REMARKABLE REFRAME: I CAN TURN PAIN INTO PURPOSE

There's just one element that makes my story different from yours, and it's who my husband is to this world. That's the only reason Bruce's situation has been able to garner mass attention and traction. Strip that away, and I am no different from you. Truth be told, I prefer to be behind the scenes, but my motivation to help others has become bigger than my desire to stay in my comfort zone.

Recently, I came across the term "helper's high," which describes that sense of fulfillment and happiness we experience when we give back. There's also research that shows that acts of kindness can boost endorphins and reduce stress. Once I understood this, my desire to give back made perfect sense. I realized that every time I opened up and shared our story, or offered support to another caregiver, I felt lighter, not because the weight of our situation lessened, but because helping others added meaning to it. There is a certain high that comes with supporting someone else. That sense of happiness feels like a gift, and I find myself embracing it more and more because, honestly, I can use all the endorphin boosts I can get!

Giving back has become part of how I cope. It shifts the focus from what's been taken from us to what I can offer in return. In many ways, sharing our story has been healing for me, and if it helps someone else along the way, then it's worth stepping outside of my comfort zone to use my voice and platform. Especially because it's something Bruce has always done.

In 1995, he founded the Willis Foundation to support youth services and education with a focus on empowering children and providing scholarships to those aging out of the foster care system. As a result, President George W. Bush appointed him the national spokesman for children in foster care in July 2002. He helped launch adoptuskids.org, a national initiative connecting waiting children with adoptive families. Bruce also believed deeply in honoring and uplifting veterans. In 2002, he purchased twelve thousand boxes of Girl Scout cookies from his daughter Tallulah (talk about winning Girl Scouts that year!) and sent them to sailors aboard the USS *John F. Kennedy* and troops in the Middle East, a small gesture to remind them of home. Then in 2003, as part of a USO tour, he traveled to Iraq with his band, the Accelerators, performing to boost morale among troops stationed overseas. This commitment extended to injured veterans, too. He participated in a television campaign for the Wounded Warrior Project, advocating for public support to assist veterans in their recovery and transition back to civilian life. Bruce's actions were driven by a quiet conviction that standing up for those without a voice could spark meaningful change.

Having learned from the best, I have found a new purpose, admittedly one I never would have gone looking for, around something that feels so painful. That is the reframe.

Through the Association for Frontotemporal Degeneration (AFTD), I get to join forces with other advocates and be of service to this community. When what I share about our family's journey gets press attention,

I know that there are thousands of untold stories just like mine, each of them deserving of compassion and concern. When I hear from another family affected by FTD or another form of dementia, I hear our story of grief, loss, and immense sadness echoed. It's important to me to be an advocate on behalf of those families who don't have the time, energy, or resources to advocate for themselves.

As hard as it was to publicly share Bruce's FTD diagnosis, I felt a calling to go beyond our family's statement, to raise my voice to bring awareness to this and other neurodegenerative diseases. I didn't want FTD to write our story, I wanted to write it. I've seen people do this for important causes and illnesses close to their hearts, and the changes that have followed have been remarkable. For instance, the Michael J. Fox Foundation has raised over $2.5 billion for research into Parkinson's, another type of neurodegenerative disease, since its founding in 2000. The foundation's efforts have led to groundbreaking advancements, including identifying key biomarkers and driving forward treatments that bring us closer to a cure. It's a powerful example of what can happen when people come together with purpose and determination. It's something Bruce always did and that has inspired me to build upon his already impactful legacy.

I want people to know that FTD is out there so that if they notice changes in their loved ones, no matter how old they are, they may feel empowered with knowledge to talk to their doctor. I want to raise awareness about all neurodegenerative diseases to increase early detection so that people spend less time without a diagnosis or with the wrong diagnosis, which can ruin families and relationships, and so they have a better chance of accessing clinical trials that could change the trajectory of their loved ones' illnesses.

Another goal is to help reduce the stigma associated with dementia. FTD is sometimes referred to as frontotemporal *degeneration*, while others call it frontotemporal *dementia*. "Degeneration" is accurate, as this disease causes parts of the frontotemporal region of the brain to degenerate. However, one challenge with using "dementia" is that many people automatically associate it with Alzheimer's and memory loss, whereas FTD presents differently. There are also varying opinions within the community about using "dementia" as a general term. Many feel it creates a picture of only the later stages of the disease and misses when the person has early symptoms and is still very active and engaged. I prefer to say "dementia" because I want to normalize the use of the word and thereby reduce the power it holds to invoke stigma. Explore and learn more about the terms "dementia" vs. "degeneration" and see what lands and feels right for you. There is no wrong answer.

People often approach me to say thank you for sharing Bruce's diagnosis. What I realized is that sharing our story has helped others feel validated and less alone when they tell their families and friends, "My loved one has what Bruce Willis has." It's as if putting a recognizable face to this disease gives them permission to speak up, seek help, and share their experiences more openly. When we share, we build connection and understanding, and that's how we start to normalize dementia and lift the burden of silence so many families carry. My hope is that eventually people will naturally have compassion and understanding for those who are diagnosed with FTD, or any form of dementia, and their care partners, without having to use Bruce's name. But if FTD becomes known as Bruce Willis's disease the way that ALS is known as Lou Gehrig's disease, and if that attention elevates research, funding, and treatment and helps the next care partner, I'm at peace with that. I know

Bruce would be, too. This will be part of his incredible legacy, one that's different than we expected, for our daughters and the world.

I also want to help reduce the stigma around caregiving and change the narrative around this really, *really* hard and heartbreaking job. For example, there is this misconception that needing outside help, such as professional caregivers, means you've "failed" in your role as a family member or partner. This stigma can prevent people from seeking support. Or too often, I see caregivers pitting themselves against one another, comparing their care to what someone else might be doing for their loved one. *Are they doing more? Am I doing enough? I would never do that to my loved one.* These comparisons and judgments can breed unnecessary guilt and shame instead of creating the support and connection we so desperately need. The truth is, every caregiving journey is unique, shaped by the individual needs of your loved one, your family dynamics, and your own capacity; no two situations are the same. There is not *just* one way to caregive or be a care partner. It's critical that we stop measuring ourselves against others and instead focus on uplifting one another. This is how we build community and recognize that we're all doing our best in an impossible situation, one we would have never dreamed of.

Along those lines, I want to help raise awareness that caregiving is not just a personal responsibility, it is a societal one, and it's essential for our government to invest in those who provide care. The emotional, physical, and financial toll of care partnership is immense. This is especially the case with FTD and other young-onset dementias because they strike people in their forties and fifties, which can be peak income-earning years. As a result, it disrupts financial stability in ways that few can prepare for, especially if you have young kids. So we need better support systems for care partners, reform in Medicare policies, and legislative change at the state and federal levels to ensure care partners have access to vital resources. The care economy in this country is an essential infrastructure that demands greater investment and attention. Caregiving shouldn't leave anyone feeling isolated or overwhelmed, because care is not just a personal duty but a collective responsibility. We need to elect leaders who recognize this reality and prioritize policies that support caregivers and families.

I am committed to using my voice to raise awareness for caregivers, brain health, and dementia because I believe action, education, and open conversation spark change. There's something powerful about thinking big, about having a goal that feels larger than yourself. It creates hope and momentum, even on the hardest days. For me, it's a way to turn pain into purpose, to make meaning out of a journey that has been so difficult. Knowing that even one caregiver might feel seen or supported makes the effort worthwhile.

There are many ways to reframe your pain into purpose in this journey, whether it's by volunteering with or donating to an organization dedicated to your loved one's disease, helping a new caregiver find resources, or sharing your journey with others via a blog, op-ed, website, or social media.

I also want to do this in order to teach my girls the most important lesson, one Bruce wanted them to learn: that even in the face of hardship, we can choose how we respond. We can let it break us, or we can use it as fuel to help ourselves and others. I don't believe that my causes or Bruce's need to become theirs, but I hope that by witnessing this work, they will carry forward a sense of empathy, resilience, and the understanding that even in our hardest moments, we still have the power to make a difference.

## REMARKABLE REFRAME:
## MY TRAUMA CAN BECOME MY
## FUEL TO SEE A BETTER DAY

I have experienced a few traumatic moments on this FTD journey, but one with deep roots occurred at our diagnosis appointment. As I've mentioned before, being sent away with a "Check back in a few months" and nothing else was so painful, scary, and yes, traumatic, that it has left a lasting imprint on me as well as a desire to prevent that moment for others if I can.

What I realized as I shared my story was that I'm not the only one who has been through this. Patients and their caregivers being sent away with nothing seems to be the norm. My experience prompted an initial call with Dr. Bruce Miller at UCSF, whom you heard from earlier in this book. I suggested creating a simple one-page road map for caregivers, and he welcomed the idea. (Of course he did; Dr. Bruce Miller is one of the most caring and thoughtful doctors I've met within the FTD space.)

Physicians typically don't have a lot of time with their patients and caregivers, so I felt that it was vital to include a list of key resources. Nothing too overwhelming—just enough so that the caregiver knows there is help and support for them. I want them to walk away with something tangible so they don't have to search the internet—especially when they don't even know what they are looking for. The one-sheet allows them to take what is relevant in the moment and leave the rest until it's needed. It can be that first navigation point on their unexpected journey.

My hope is that more doctors and their offices will follow suit and compile this type of road map. Caregivers already walk into the diagnosis with their hands full. Hopefully, this will take one thing off their list.

I know that I already shared this story about leaving our diagnosis appointment with nothing, but if something good can come from it, then it's important for me to focus on that. My trauma has become my fuel to see a better day for myself and others. Eventually, I hope your trauma becomes fuel for something positive, too.

## ONE THING TO CONSIDER . . .

One way to turn pain into purpose is to consider brain donation after your loved one passes away. This is another area that I am passionate about, and yet I know it's a sensitive topic. Many of us check the box on our driver's license to become organ donors, a noble and beautiful act that can save lives. However, brain donation is a separate process and serves a different purpose: It advances critical research to better understand, treat, and hopefully cure neurodegenerative diseases like FTD, Alzheimer's, and Parkinson's.

According to Bill Seeley, MD, professor of neurology and pathology at the UCSF Memory and Aging Center and director of the UCSF Neurodegenerative Disease Brain Bank, there are many reasons to consider this.

- **Emotional closure for you as the care partner and for your family.** This is especially the case when your person's diagnosis can't be confirmed while they are alive.

"The brain autopsy settles the issue once and for all, can help you make sense of the symptoms and put a specific label on the problem," says Seeley. "For some people, that knowledge helps them feel more settled that there was nothing else to be done. For others it gives them a more specific target for their advocacy and for others still it becomes a matter of family planning and counseling if, for example, a heritable disease is identified."

- **A sense of legacy.** "After battling a disease for so long, caregivers know better than anyone the toll that these diseases can take on the human spirit. Many express a desire to do anything they can to help prevent others from having to experience such a hardship," says Seeley. "Brain donation is a positive, affirming step a caregiver can take to make a difference in the race to uncover new treatments and preventions for dementia. Even the patient himself or herself may take comfort in the gesture if their cognitive status allows."

- **A contribution to science.** The benefits of brain donation to science and society are not hypothetical or academic; they are concrete and impactful.

  "Most of the major therapeutic targets being pursued by the pharmaceutical industry today, including those that gave rise to recently approved Alzheimer's disease treatments, were identified through the study of human brain tissue donated by patients," says Seeley. "Without the fundamental information that we gain by studying brain tissue, we just can't know what a disease really is."

Katie Brandt of the Frontotemporal Disorders Unit at Massachusetts General Hospital, who was a caregiver for her husband who passed away from FTD, adds, "The gift of brain donation is to forever have your voice be a part of the story of unlocking the secrets of FTD and curing it."

If you're interested in brain donation, a good place to start is by speaking with your neurologist, as they can help navigate the local logistics. If they aren't familiar with the process, national resources like the Brain Donor Project can provide guidance and information. Learn more at braindonorproject.org.

OUR CAREGIVING EXPERIENCE will shift our perspective on life. While it can feel like a horrible nightmare, I promise that there is meaning and purpose to be found. I didn't realize that in the early days, and no one told me otherwise, which is why I feel it's important to share this with you now. For some, this journey may spark a sense of purpose or a calling to give back in some way. But I also want to acknowledge that many may not have the time, energy, or capacity to seek meaning while in the thick of caregiving, and that's okay. Please know that you have others in your corner who see you, stand with you, and are lifting you up. If and when you are ready, you may find the capacity to join us. Our lives can feel fuller with more meaning and color when we're open to allowing that in, recognizing that both the positive and the painful can coexist. I have decided to accept what is and seek out the beauty in this new chapter. I hope you can, in your own time, too.

*Something to think about . . .*

What is one small reframe you can make about your journey?

_____

_____

_____

_____

_____

_____

_____

_____

_____

_____

_____

_____

_____

_____

_____

_____

_____

_____

# Conclusion

Recently, Mabel wanted to take me on a mommy-daughter date to see the musical *Hamilton*. I thought, *Oh boy, a three-hour show?* Evelyn, ever her father's child, said, "Three hours? I'll sit this one out. You guys go have some fun," flashing Bruce's signature smirk at me.

Early in my relationship with Bruce, knowing I wasn't a big Broadway buff, he gave me permission to skip any show that ran longer than ninety minutes. He'd say, "Stick to the one-acts, Em." Still, there are things we'll happily do for our children. As Mabel and I settled into our seats, I exhaled, grateful for the simple fact that I could sit there for three hours, knowing Bruce was safe and cared for. I could rest easy. I muted my Apple Watch, silencing the alerts and reminders tied to our second home, allowing myself to be fully present with Mabel, who wanted this time with me. Not that long ago, moments like this were impossible.

Oddly enough, I looked over and noticed another primary caregiver I follow on Instagram sitting in the audience, too. She had recently lost her mother to Alzheimer's, and I couldn't help but wonder if she was slowly trying to reclaim parts of her life as well.

Before becoming a caregiver, I took so much for granted; the ease of daily life, the spontaneity, and the freedom to fully immerse myself in the present. Now, as a navigator in this journey, I see that some color has been brought back into our world. The reframe has been in recognizing just how lucky the girls and I are to reclaim even small parts of our lives, not all of it, but enough. And those parts are met with so much joy, gratitude, and enthusiasm. Our lives will never be the same, and as much as I grieve this experience daily, as I know so many other caregivers do, I can also sit here and tell you we are better for it.

Prior to seeing *Hamilton*, I wish someone had given me a heads-up that I'd need more than water and a snack to get through the show; I'd also need one of Bruce's handkerchiefs, because I bawled my eyes out more than once. Thankfully the woman next to me was prepared and offered me a tissue as we wept together. A few songs hit me hard, but the one that sent me over the edge was "Who Lives, Who Dies, Who Tells Your Story."

The final song is a reflection on legacy, memory, and the impact a person's life can have long after they're gone. The song explores the idea that even great achievements and lives can fade unless someone actively steps up to preserve and share those stories. After Alexander Hamilton's death, his wife, Eliza, takes on the role of storyteller, dedicating herself to preserving his legacy, building institutions, and advocating for the causes he believed in.

It made me think of caregivers. Could this be our theme song? We carry the stories of our loved ones, becoming their voices when they can no longer share their own. Just as Eliza Hamilton stepped forward to preserve Alexander's legacy, caregivers step into that space, ensuring that the essence of who our person was isn't erased or distilled down to just their disease.

That line *Who tells your story?* has echoed in my mind long after the curtain call. As caregivers, we ask ourselves the same question. *Are we doing enough? Are we honoring our loved one properly?* We don't just handle appointments, medications, and routines. We hold on to memories, safeguard our loved one's dignity, and fiercely protect who they were before dementia.

Bruce's story will continue. His legacy will live on through our family, his work in film and music, and the millions of lives he's touched. But I believe he's leaving something even more profound, something that will ripple far beyond Hollywood. His journey is shaping the conversation around FTD, dementia, and caregiving, shifting the narrative in ways I hope will soften the experience for others walking this path.

I know Bruce's legacy won't just be about the art he created; it will be about how he loved and how that love carries on through us. And as I sat in the theater, with Mabel by my side, I realized I'm not just telling his story. Just like Eliza, I'm committed to continuing it.

No matter where you are in this journey, know this: Color *will* return. It may not look the same, but it will be beautiful in its own way. Applaud yourself for the work you're doing, one of the hardest jobs in the world. Your loved one would be proud. Not just for the care you've given, but for the way you're honoring them by continuing to tell their story and for how you are choosing to show up for yourself.

# ACKNOWLEDGMENTS

As I began writing these acknowledgments, I quickly realized what a daunting task it would be. The truth is, I don't want to leave anyone out. Our family has been held in so much love by longtime friends, family, and the incredible people I've brought into our circle to help support us who now feel like extended family. Our village has wrapped their arms around us. They check in on Bruce, they show up for our children, and they show up for me. I'm eternally grateful to each and every one of them.

First and foremost, I want to acknowledge my husband, Bruce.

I still can't quite believe this is the book I ended up writing, or the life I've had to become an expert in. Something about that feels profoundly tragic. Bruce's illness changed everything. And yet, from that grief and unraveling came something that has transformed me at my core.

How do you thank the person whose struggle has so deeply shaped your path? I hate this for him. I would change it all in a heartbeat. But I can't and, boy, have I tried. So I have to live in what is, and find the grace in it.

I'm grateful Bruce walked into my life. He made me a better human, a more compassionate one. And I love him so deeply for who he is now, for who he was, and for everything we still are together.

To my mother, Zorina: You've always shown me what it means to care deeply and be there for the people you love. Your strength and grace have been my greatest teachers. I'm so grateful we get to do this life together. Thank you for being my constant, for being there for your granddaughters and son-in-law, who has always felt a loving connection to you. Loves, Mom.

To my daughters, Mabel and Evelyn: Thank you for cheering me on in this effort to help others, even when it meant I had less free time to be with you. You understood the importance of what I was trying to do and encouraged me to keep going. You've reminded me to be vulnerable and always stay in truth. When you said, "Mom, this will help people," that's all I needed to keep putting one foot in front of the other. I love you both so much.

To my stepdaughters, Rumer, Scout, and Tallulah: You are pure love. To be in your orbit is a privilege. You show up for me and your younger sisters in ways that are so beautiful and pure. I'm so fortunate to know you and even luckier to call you family. Thank you for all your love, encouragement, and support. I adore you.

To Demi: You have always been a trusted, honest sounding board. I'm endlessly grateful for the way you've reimagined and redefined what family can look like. What you and Bruce created laid the foundation for all of us—it truly set us up for success. Thank you.

To Bruce's family. To my mother-in-law, Marlena: Thank you for offering your steady love and support. To David and Flo: I'm lucky to call you my brother- and sister-in-law. The kindness and care that you, your spouses, and your children exude is something we all feel and truly appreciate. And to Bruce's cousins and extended family, Marci, Nita, Sharon, Ed, and Ronna: Thank you for continuing to show up for Bruce. It warms my heart more than words can express.

To Bruce's core crew: Stephen Eads, who has been our constant through thick and thin—I couldn't have done so much of this without your care and support of Bruce and our family. And to Lori A., Glenn C., John C., David G., Doug H., Robert and Beth K., Bruce and Sue Ann L., Kevin and Rose M., Johnny M., John M., M. Night S., Sheri S., Chris S., Lori S., Adam P., Gunnar P., Arnold R., Hunter R., and Stuart W.: Your love for Bruce and the way you've been a source of support for our family has been one of the greatest gifts I've been able to witness. Thank you for being there in ways big and small. We've felt every bit of it.

To my literary agents, Mollie Glick and Anthony Mattero: Thank you for believing in me and recognizing that I had something to say, even before I could fully see it myself. Writing a book was never something I dreamed of or had on my bucket list, but it has become one of the most rewarding experiences of my life. Thank you for guiding me through all the steps of this new journey. It's been a privilege to do this with you.

To Maria Shriver: My mentor, friend, and daily source of inspiration. You believed in and trusted me to take this abstract idea and shape it into something real. Writing this book has brought me healing in ways I didn't expect, and I'll forever be grateful for the lifeline you threw me.

To my editors at The Open Field, Meg Leder and Nina Rodríguez-Marty: Thank you for the care, thoughtfulness, and heart you brought to every page. Your feedback, ideas, and edits helped shape this book into exactly what it needed to be: a guide to caring for the caregiver. I truly loved working with you both and wish I could write ten more books just to keep going with you.

To my collaborator, Michele Bender: The person I had the privilege of spending the most time with during this journey. From day one, you championed this book and its purpose with unwavering commitment. You've been my cheerleader, my partner, and my steady hand as I found my voice and courage as a new writer. I always felt seen and supported by you. I loved how in sync we were, how seamlessly we worked together. Your dedication helped this book take root and bloom into *The Unexpected Journey*. Thank you, Michele.

To Norman Jean Roy: Thank you for capturing our family with such beauty and tenderness at every stage of our lives. The cover photo is no exception; it's another stunning reflection of your gift. I'm so grateful for you, Jojo, and your girls, who were born around the same time as ours. Knowing that your work graces the cover of this book makes it that much sweeter. We love you so.

I feel incredibly fortunate to have both my own circle of trusted business advisers and those I've inherited through Bruce, who care for and protect us with all their might. Their loyalty and commitment mean everything.

To Ben Rubinfeld: Thank you for looking out for me during this process and beyond, and for your steady guidance. To Marty Singer: Thank you for being the bulldog that you are and a constant source of strength and protection.

To Paul Zukowsky: You've been more than a business manager for twenty-five-plus years; you've become someone I turn to for guidance in every area of my life. I'm so grateful to know you. You are family. Sara S., Jessica S., Tracy S., Jessica M., and the rest of the ML Management team: Your work and dedication to our family has never gone unnoticed.

To Lauren Kucerak, my publicist and friend for twenty-five years: You have been a fierce protector and my biggest supporter, constantly pushing me forward and believing in me. I'm so deeply thankful for you.

To Sam Mast, Bruce's longtime publicist: Thank you for holding our family's hand through this journey. You've been an anchor and a sounding board, always keeping Bruce's protection front and center. I'm so grateful you're in our lives. To Alan Nierob for looking out for us. Thank you for your guidance and help. And I just have to take a moment for Paul Bloch: You were the greatest protector and friend to Bruce from day one. I wish you were still here walking alongside us and guiding us. Paul, we miss you dearly.

To Kathy Gordon: Thank you for your expertise and strategy in getting this book into the right hands.

To The Open Field: Brian Tart, Allison Dobson, Anna Brill, Jason Ramirez, Bridget Gilleran, Anna Dobbin, Nick Michal, Christina Nguyen, and Susan VanHecke, I'm honored to be in your professional and capable hands.

To Shelby Meizlik: Thank you for your guidance, thoughtful strategy, and unwavering belief in this book. Your dedication has helped bring this message into the world with heart and impact.

To the CAA team: You've been nothing short of terrific. To Bianca Petcu: Thank you for your trusted legal guidance. To Agnès Rigou for helping get the book translated so it can reach caregivers around the world. And to Via Romano and Sydney Shiffman: Thank you for your professionalism and support.

To my friends and community who have held me up, been there to listen, let me cry, laughed with me, checked in on us, cheered me on, and held my hand, thank you for being there and showing up for me and my family: Ricky A., Mary Jo B., Jill C., Jody C., Dennis C., Ingrid C., Helen and Tim C., Kerry and Pete C. and their sweet boys for keeping Mr. Bruce and our family in their prayers, Allison and Keith C., Serene C., Patti D., Nancy E., Stevee Jo E., Britta F., Anne F., Amanda G., Brandi G., Franne G., Melisa and Alan G., Mike G., Patti H., Red H., Linde J., Ali K., Donna K., Michael K., Anne Cutbill L., Quoc M., Kathleen M., Mary Louise P., Tracy P., Keith R., Sujean R., Jane R., Laura S., Chelsea S., Abby S., Allyn S., Dr. S., Bita T., Carmela T., Kristen and Josh T., and Juliya and Ari S.

To the Village School staff who always had a watchful eye on our girls, and also to Annie B., Yvette D., John E., and Kathy S.

To my extended family at AFTD and especially to those who wrapped their arms around me and our family when we needed it most.

To Susan Dickinson, who sensed trouble in the waters before I even knew what was happening: Your love and care have been a steady anchor. Thank you for offering us a safe place to land and the security we've so deeply needed on this journey. I admire you and all that you continue to do for the FTD community.

To Ben Freeman, who helped me find my footing in those early, shaky days when I wasn't even sure I had a voice strong enough to speak up: Thank you for helping me begin to use it.

To Kristin Holloway, my first connection to another FTD family walking a similar path with a young child: You opened my eyes to the possibility of different avenues of care and reminded me that it's possible to raise young children with grace and strength in the midst of it all. Thank you.

To Sharon Denny, whose generous and kind heart I've had the privilege of learning from: It's a gift to witness the support and compassion you extend not only to me and our family but our whole FTD community. Thank you.

To David Pfeifer, who generously shared his story of caregiving while raising his boys: Thank you for always being just a call or text away.

To Gail Andersen, who reached out in those early days: Hearing how you navigated this path while raising your own children gave me strength and the hope that my girls would be okay, too.

To Meghan Buzby, Penny Dacks, Bridget Graham, Esther Kane, PJ Lepp, Kathy Newhouse Mele, Don Newhouse, Matthew Sharp, and Phillip Weichel: Thank you for the ways you've each shown up.

To Senator Michelle Hinchey: Thank you for the awareness and attention you've brought to FTD, and for the incredible work you've done in New York. Watching you champion real change has been so moving and inspiring. Your leadership gives me hope and has encouraged me to use my voice.

To Elizabeth Ashford: Thank you for helping me find my advocacy voice. You've had the patience to teach me about policy and legislation, everything I must've missed in fifth grade! I hope you can hear echoes of your voice in these pages. You've shaped me more than you know.

To Sara M.: You have turned over every stone for Bruce and our family, again and again. Most of all, you helped me return to my role as Bruce's wife. I'm forever grateful to you.

To our Private Health Management team: Megan G., Kristin L., Zoe M., and Jimmy W.: Thank you for being the dream team that brought stability back into our lives. You surrounded us with the level of care we needed to keep going.

To the Motion Picture & Television Fund: Thank you for giving Bruce and me a safe place to land while I navigate the beautiful and complex world of palliative care. My heartfelt gratitude to Angela C., Jessica C., Anne F., Linda H., Daniel K., Tiffany L., Arthur R., Wilson W., and Veronica Z.

To the team that surrounds our family with love and unwavering support: Grant A., Dr. Linus A., Jun A., Alfredo M., Rachel A., Megan A., Veronica B., Victor B. along with Fergus and Frodo, Dr. Zachary B., Alyssa C., Dr. Anthony C., Danielle C., Dr. Marvin C., Curtis C., Kate C., Josh D., Michele E., Dylan F., Mateo F., Kirk G., Dr. Jeffery G., Ryan G., Yesenia G., Andrew H., Barbara H., Lety H., Linda H., Suzannah H., Dr. Richard I., Dr. Sheldon J., Tara J., Jay K., Mihae K., Dr. Sarah K., Ana M., Dr. Bruce M., Bobo M., Dr. David M., Ezekiel M., Dr. Mario M., Ryan M., Gabby M.,

Dr. John O., Chris P., Nissa P., Ruthie P., Dr. Chris R., Erica R., Anthony S., Dr. Abdi S., Dave S., Raja S., Teepa S., Wendy S., Ursula T., Heidi W., November W., Dr. Sherry Y., Veronica V., and Bruce's amazing team of medical advisers and providers.

To all the contributors and experts who lent their voices and wisdom to this book: Thank you for guiding me, and for lighting the path for the next caregiver who comes along. A special thank-you as well to Polly L. and Anil V. for your steady presence.

To you, the person holding this book in your hands: Thank you for trusting me with your time. I hope something in these pages has offered you comfort, clarity, or companionship. Writing this helped me heal parts of my journey, and my hope is that reading it does the same for you. Make time.

And to Bruce's incredible, unwavering fans: Thank you for loving him, for holding him in your hearts, and for keeping our family in your prayers. Witnessing the depth of love and admiration for him has been profoundly moving. It's a gift I do not take for granted and nor did he.